Recent Advances in Pneumonia in Older People

Recent Advances in Pneumonia in Older People

Editors

Satoru Ebihara
Takae Ebihara

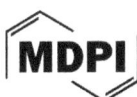

Basel • Beijing • Wuhan • Barcelona • Belgrade • Novi Sad • Cluj • Manchester

Editors
Satoru Ebihara
Department of Internal
Medicine and Rehabilitation
Science
Tohoku University Graduate
School of Medicine
Sendai, Japan

Takae Ebihara
Department of Geriatric
Medicine
Kyorin University School of
Medicine
Tokyo, Japan

Editorial Office
MDPI
St. Alban-Anlage 66
4052 Basel, Switzerland

This is a reprint of articles from the Special Issue published online in the open access journal *Journal of Clinical Medicine* (ISSN 2077-0383) (available at: https://www.mdpi.com/journal/jcm/special_issues/Pneumonia_Older).

For citation purposes, cite each article independently as indicated on the article page online and as indicated below:

Lastname, A.A.; Lastname, B.B. Article Title. *Journal Name* **Year**, *Volume Number*, Page Range.

ISBN 978-3-0365-9851-2 (Hbk)
ISBN 978-3-0365-9852-9 (PDF)
doi.org/10.3390/books978-3-0365-9852-9

© 2024 by the authors. Articles in this book are Open Access and distributed under the Creative Commons Attribution (CC BY) license. The book as a whole is distributed by MDPI under the terms and conditions of the Creative Commons Attribution-NonCommercial-NoDerivs (CC BY-NC-ND) license.

Contents

About the Editors vii

Satoru Ebihara, Tatsuma Okazaki, Keisuke Obata and Takae Ebihara
Importance of Skeletal Muscle and Interdisciplinary Team Approach in Managing Pneumonia in Older People
Reprinted from: *J. Clin. Med.* **2023**, *12*, 5093, doi:10.3390/jcm12155093 1

Nanako Shiokawa, Tatsuma Okazaki, Yoshimi Suzukamo, Midori Miyatake, Mana Kogure, Naoki Nakaya, et al.
Association between Low Forced Vital Capacity and High Pneumonia Mortality, and Impact of Muscle Power
Reprinted from: *J. Clin. Med.* **2023**, *12*, 3272, doi:10.3390/jcm12093272 4

Yuki Yoshimatsu, Masaharu Aga, Kosaku Komiya, Shusaku Haranaga, Yuka Numata, Makoto Miki, et al.
The Clinical Significance of Anaerobic Coverage in the Antibiotic Treatment of Aspiration Pneumonia: A Systematic Review and Meta-Analysis
Reprinted from: *J. Clin. Med.* **2023**, *12*, 1992, doi:10.3390/jcm12051992 14

Ryo Ichibayashi, Hideki Sekiya, Kosuke Kaneko and Mitsuru Honda
Use of Maximum Tongue Pressure Values to Examine the Presence of Dysphagia after Extubation and Prevent Aspiration Pneumonia in Elderly Emergency Patients
Reprinted from: *J. Clin. Med.* **2022**, *11*, 6599, doi:10.3390/jcm11216599 25

Camilla Koch Ryrsø, Arnold Matovu Dungu, Maria Hein Hegelund, Daniel Faurholt-Jepsen, Bente Klarlund Pedersen, Christian Ritz, et al.
Physical Inactivity and Sedentarism during and after Admission with Community-Acquired Pneumonia and the Risk of Readmission and Mortality: A Prospective Cohort Study
Reprinted from: *J. Clin. Med.* **2022**, *11*, 5923, doi:10.3390/jcm11195923 36

Yuki Yoshimatsu and David G. Smithard
A Paradigm Shift in the Diagnosis of Aspiration Pneumonia in Older Adults
Reprinted from: *J. Clin. Med.* **2022**, *11*, 5214, doi:10.3390/jcm11175214 48

Takae Ebihara
Comprehensive Approaches to Aspiration Pneumonia and Dysphagia in the Elderly on the Disease Time-Axis
Reprinted from: *J. Clin. Med.* **2022**, *11*, 5323, doi:10.3390/jcm11185323 64

Midori Miyatake, Tatsuma Okazaki, Yoshimi Suzukamo, Sanae Matsuyama, Ichiro Tsuji and Shin-Ichi Izumi
High Mortality in an Older Japanese Population with Low Forced Vital Capacity and Gender-Dependent Potential Impact of Muscle Strength: Longitudinal Cohort Study
Reprinted from: *J. Clin. Med.* **2022**, *11*, 5264, doi:10.3390/jcm11185264 78

Ikuko Okuni and Satoru Ebihara
Are Oropharyngeal Dysphagia Screening Tests Effective in Preventing Pneumonia?
Reprinted from: *J. Clin. Med.* **2022**, *11*, 370, doi:10.3390/jcm11020370 88

Anja Maria Raab, Gabi Mueller, Simone Elsig, Simon C. Gandevia, Marcel Zwahlen, Maria T. E. Hopman and Roger Hilfiker
Systematic Review of Incidence Studies of Pneumonia in Persons with Spinal Cord Injury
Reprinted from: *J. Clin. Med.* **2022**, *11*, 211, doi:10.3390/jcm11010211 100

Lucía Méndez, Pedro Castro, Jorge Ferreira and Cátia Caneiras
Epidemiological Characterization and the Impact of Healthcare-Associated Pneumonia in Patients Admitted in a Northern Portuguese Hospital
Reprinted from: *J. Clin. Med.* **2021**, *10*, 5593, doi:10.3390/jcm10235593 . . . . **118**

About the Editors

Satoru Ebihara

Satoru Ebihara graduated from Tohoku University School of Medicine in 1990 and trained at Tohoku University Hospital, McGill University, and Toho University. His research interests range from aspiration pneumonia to dyspnea sensations in various settings. Recently, he has used multi-omics analysis to explore the fundamental mechanisms of dyspnea sensations.

Takae Ebihara

Geriatrician. Having graduated from Akita University School of Medicine in 1990, she worked on the pathogenesis of aspiration pneumonia as pioneering member of the Dept. of Geriatrics and Respiratory Medicine at Tohoku Univ. In 1996–2000, she engaged in research on lung mechanics at Meakins–Christie Labs, McGill Univ., Canada, as a post-doctoral fellow. In 2000–2014, she returned to Tohoku Univ. to explore the pathogenesis of aspiration pneumonia and its unique prevention as an Assistant Professor in the Dept. of Geriatrics and Gerontology. Since 2016, she has engaged in clinical practice, research, and medical education as an Associate Professor in the Dept. of Geriatrics at Kyorin University in Tokyo. Thanks to her experience, she has received the Tohoku University Gender Equality Award (Sawayanagi Prize) for promoting a sustainable work–life balance. She is also active in diversity promotion activities.

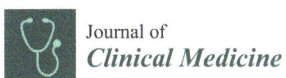

Editorial

Importance of Skeletal Muscle and Interdisciplinary Team Approach in Managing Pneumonia in Older People

Satoru Ebihara [1,*], Tatsuma Okazaki [1], Keisuke Obata [1] and Takae Ebihara [2]

1. Department of Internal Medicine and Rehabilitation Science, Tohoku University Graduate School of Medicine, Sendai 980-8574, Japan; tmokazaki0808@gmail.com (T.O.); keisuke.obata1110@gmail.com (K.O.)
2. Department of Geriatric Medicine, Graduate School of Medicine, Kyorin University, Tokyo 181-8611, Japan; takae–u.ac.jp
* Correspondence: satoru.ebihara.c4@tohoku.ac.jp; Tel.: +81-22-717-7353

Pneumonia is the most frequent lower respiratory tract disease and a major cause of morbidity and mortality globally [1]. Several attempts have been made to categorize it based on origin, clinical setting in which the patient contracts it, and pattern of lung parenchyma involvement, and others. The classification of pneumonia is becoming more complex with the increasing diversity of patient populations.

The most common classification of pneumonia is based on the location where pneumonia occur. Community-acquired pneumonia occur at the community and hospital-acquired pneumonia occur at the hospital. Pneumonia among residents of nursing homes or long-term care facilities is categorized as nursing-home-acquired pneumonia. This concept is based on the idea that the causative bacterium of pneumonia is determined to some extent by the location where pneumonia occur and serves as a guideline for the use of antibiotics [2–4]. Guidelines have been established for each type of pneumonia. However, deaths from pneumonia have continued to increase annually with the population aging, even after the publication of these guidelines [1]. This indicates that the guidelines for pneumonia treatment should not only be focused on the use of antibiotics.

Aspiration pneumonia is the most dominant form of pneumonia in older adults [5]. Many studies have been conducted on dysphagia, aspiration, and countermeasures. However, not all cases of aspiration result in pneumonia, and the development of pneumonia involves several steps, such as coughing, spitting, cilia in the airways, handling foreign bodies in the airways, and immunity [6]. Few studies have discussed countermeasures linking aspiration to pneumonia. In this special issue, six original studies and four review articles can be found that provide new insights into pneumonia in older people.

Serial studies concerning the relationship between forced vital capacity (FVC) on spirometry and death due to pneumonia in older people have been published by the same laboratory in Japan. In the first study, the authors analyzed the data of a large cohort and found that low FVC was associated with a high all-cause mortality rate of community-dwelling older people [7]. In the second study, the authors reported a stronger relationship between FVC and pneumonia mortality than between FVC and all-cause mortality [8]. They suggested the involvement of impaired leg muscle strength in pneumonia-related deaths. In addition, researchers in Denmark reported that physical inactivity and sedation during and after admission of older patients with aspiration pneumonia were related to mortality [9]. Ichibayashi et al. showed that the maximum tongue pressure after extubation can predict post-extubation aspiration pneumonia in older patients receiving mechanical ventilation [10].

Taken together, the above four reports indicate a strong relationship between impairment of skeletal muscle and pneumonia or pneumonia-related death of older adults. Mendes and colleagues showed that healthcare-associated pneumonia is the main causes of hospital admission and death among patients with pneumonia, the majority of which

Citation: Ebihara, S.; Okazaki, T.; Obata, K.; Ebihara, T. Importance of Skeletal Muscle and Interdisciplinary Team Approach in Managing Pneumonia in Older People. *J. Clin. Med.* **2023**, *12*, 5093. https://doi.org/10.3390/jcm12155093

Received: 26 July 2023
Accepted: 1 August 2023
Published: 3 August 2023

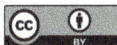

Copyright: © 2023 by the authors. Licensee MDPI, Basel, Switzerland. This article is an open access article distributed under the terms and conditions of the Creative Commons Attribution (CC BY) license (https://creativecommons.org/licenses/by/4.0/).

were empirically treated, in Portugal [11]. The high frailty ratio of patients with healthcare-associated pneumonia in this study also suggested a strong relationship between a decline in skeletal muscle function and pneumonia-related death. A systematic review showed that pneumonia is a clinically relevant complication in patients with spinal cord injury and prevention should be targeted at patients with tetraplegia, suggesting the importance of skeletal muscles in the development of fatal pneumonia [12].

The remaining four papers in this issue highlight the importance of comprehensive functional assessment and interdisciplinary team care, which is beyond the use of antibiotics, in older patients with aspiration pneumonia. Yoshimatsu et al. reported no evidence of the benefit of anaerobic coverage in the antibiotic treatment of aspiration pneumonia [13]. They also reported that the simplistic and knee-jerk diagnosis of aspiration pneumonia is not based on important investigations and functional assessments, resulting in inappropriate patient management [14]. These reports suggest that careful assessment plays a pivotal role in the management of aspiration pneumonia. Okuni and Ebihara showed that dysphagia screening tests, such as the water swallowing test, were useful in predicting future aspiration, and an interdisciplinary team approach may be effective in preventing aspiration pneumonia [15]. However, they could not determine what kind of team approach was most effective in preventing aspiration pneumonia in older adults. A review by Ebihara provides some hints. The review stated that the team approach to managing aspiration pneumonia differed depending on the time axis of disease progression in managing aspiration pneumonia [16].

Since this special issue reveals the importance of skeletal muscle and an interdisciplinary team approach, it will help clinicians make decisions and treatment choices. We appreciate the valuable contributions of all authors. We are also grateful to the reviewers for their professional and constructive comments and to the JCM team for their continuous support with this special issue.

Author Contributions: Conceptualization, S.E.; methodology, T.O., K.O. and T.E.; writing—original draft preparation, S.E.; writing—review and editing, T.O., K.O. and T.E. All authors have read and agreed to the published version of the manuscript.

Funding: This work was supported by the Research Funding for Longevity Sciences from the National Center for Geriatrics and Gerontology (22-1), JSPS KAKENHI (19H03984, 19K22821, and 22K19760).

Conflicts of Interest: The authors declare no conflict of interest.

References

1. Feldman, C.; Shaddock, E. Epidemiology of lower respiratory tract infections in adults. *Expert. Rev. Respir. Med.* **2019**, *13*, 63–77. [CrossRef] [PubMed]
2. Wilson, K.C.; Schoenberg, N.C.; Cohn, D.L.; Crothers, K.; Fennelly, K.P.; Metlay, J.P.; Saukkonen, J.J.; Strange, C.; Waterer, G.; Dweik, R. Community-acquired Pneumonia Guideline Recommendations-Impact of a Consensus-based Process versus Systematic Reviews. *Clin. Infect. Dis.* **2021**, *73*, e1467–e1475. [CrossRef] [PubMed]
3. Martin-Loeches, I.; Rodriguez, A.H.; Torres, A. New guidelines for hospital-acquired pneumonia/ventilator-associated pneumonia: USA vs. Europe. *Curr. Opin. Crit. Care* **2018**, *24*, 347–352. [CrossRef] [PubMed]
4. Naughton, B.J.; Mylotte, J.M. Treatment guideline for nursing home-acquired pneumonia based on community practice. *J. Am. Geriatr. Soc.* **2000**, *48*, 82–88. [CrossRef] [PubMed]
5. Teramoto, S.; Fukuchi, Y.; Sasaki, H.; Sato, K.; Sekizawa, K.; Matsuse, T. Japanese Study Group on Aspiration Pulmonary Disease. High incidence of aspiration pneumonia in community- and hospital-acquired pneumonia in hospitalized patients: A multicenter, prospective study in Japan. *J. Am. Geriatr. Soc.* **2008**, *56*, 577–579. [CrossRef] [PubMed]
6. Ebihara, S.; Sekiya, H.; Miyagi, M.; Ebihara, T.; Okazaki, T. Dysphagia, dystussia, and aspiration pneumonia in elderly people. *J. Thorac. Dis.* **2016**, *8*, 632–639. [CrossRef] [PubMed]
7. Miyatake, M.; Okazaki, T.; Suzukamo, Y.; Matsuyama, S.; Tsuji, I.; Izumi, S.I. High Mortality in an Older Japanese Population with Low Forced Vital Capacity and Gender-Dependent Potential Impact of Muscle Strength: Longitudinal Cohort Study. *J. Clin. Med.* **2022**, *11*, 5264. [CrossRef] [PubMed]
8. Shiokawa, N.; Okazaki, T.; Suzukamo, Y.; Miyatake, M.; Kogure, M.; Nakaya, N.; Hozawa, A.; Ebihara, S.; Izumi, S.I. Association between Low Forced Vital Capacity and High Pneumonia Mortality, and Impact of Muscle Power. *J. Clin. Med.* **2023**, *12*, 3272. [CrossRef] [PubMed]

9. Ryrsø, C.K.; Dungu, A.M.; Hegelund, M.H.; Faurholt-Jepsen, D.; Pedersen, B.K.; Ritz, C.; Lindegaard, B.; Krogh-Madsen, R. Physical Inactivity and Sedentarism during and after Admission with Community-Acquired Pneumonia and the Risk of Readmission and Mortality: A Prospective Cohort Study. *J. Clin. Med.* **2022**, *11*, 5923. [CrossRef] [PubMed]
10. Ichibayashi, R.; Sekiya, H.; Kaneko, K.; Honda, M. Use of Maximum Tongue Pressure Values to Examine the Presence of Dysphagia after Extubation and Prevent Aspiration Pneumonia in Elderly Emergency Patients. *J. Clin. Med.* **2022**, *11*, 6599. [CrossRef] [PubMed]
11. Méndez, L.; Castro, P.; Ferreira, J.; Caneiras, C. Epidemiological Characterization and the Impact of Healthcare-Associated Pneumonia in Patients Admitted in a Northern Portuguese Hospital. *J. Clin. Med.* **2021**, *10*, 5593. [CrossRef] [PubMed]
12. Raab, A.M.; Mueller, G.; Elsig, S.; Gandevia, S.C.; Zwahlen, M.; Hopman, M.T.E.; Hilfiker, R. Systematic Review of Incidence Studies of Pneumonia in Persons with Spinal Cord Injury. *J. Clin. Med.* **2021**, *11*, 211. [CrossRef] [PubMed]
13. Yoshimatsu, Y.; Aga, M.; Komiya, K.; Haranaga, S.; Numata, Y.; Miki, M.; Higa, F.; Senda, K.; Teramoto, S. The Clinical Significance of Anaerobic Coverage in the Antibiotic Treatment of Aspiration Pneumonia: A Systematic Review and Meta-Analysis. *J. Clin. Med.* **2023**, *12*, 1992. [CrossRef] [PubMed]
14. Yoshimatsu, Y.; Smithard, D.G. A Paradigm Shift in the Diagnosis of Aspiration Pneumonia in Older Adults. *J. Clin. Med.* **2022**, *11*, 5214. [CrossRef] [PubMed]
15. Okuni, I.; Ebihara, S. Are Oropharyngeal Dysphagia Screening Tests Effective in Preventing Pneumonia? *J. Clin. Med.* **2022**, *11*, 370. [CrossRef] [PubMed]
16. Ebihara, T. Comprehensive Approaches to Aspiration Pneumonia and Dysphagia in the Elderly on the Disease Time-Axis. *J. Clin. Med.* **2022**, *11*, 5323. [CrossRef] [PubMed]

Disclaimer/Publisher's Note: The statements, opinions and data contained in all publications are solely those of the individual author(s) and contributor(s) and not of MDPI and/or the editor(s). MDPI and/or the editor(s) disclaim responsibility for any injury to people or property resulting from any ideas, methods, instructions or products referred to in the content.

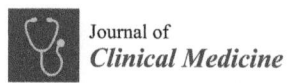

Article

Association between Low Forced Vital Capacity and High Pneumonia Mortality, and Impact of Muscle Power

Nanako Shiokawa [1], Tatsuma Okazaki [1,2,*], Yoshimi Suzukamo [1], Midori Miyatake [1], Mana Kogure [3], Naoki Nakaya [3], Atsushi Hozawa [3], Satoru Ebihara [4] and Shin-Ichi Izumi [1,2,5]

1. Department of Physical Medicine and Rehabilitation, Tohoku University Graduate School of Medicine, Sendai 980-8575, Japan
2. Center for Dysphagia, Tohoku University Hospital, Sendai 980-8574, Japan
3. Department of Preventive Medicine and Epidemiology, Tohoku Medical Megabank Organization, Sendai 980-8575, Japan
4. Department of Internal Medicine and Rehabilitation Science, Tohoku University Graduate School of Medicine, Sendai 980-8574, Japan
5. Department of Physical Medicine and Rehabilitation, Tohoku University Graduate School of Biomedical Engineering, Sendai 980-8575, Japan
* Correspondence: tmokazaki0808@gmail.com; Tel.: +81-22-717-7338

Abstract: Impaired % predicted value forced vital capacity (% FVC) is related to higher all-cause mortality in aged adults, and strong muscle force may improve this relationship. A muscle disease, sarcopenia, causes higher mortality. We aimed to identify the unknown disease that relates impaired % FVC with higher mortality in aged adults among the three major leading causes of death, and the effect of strong leg force on this relationship. Cox proportional hazard model analyzed the longitudinal Tsurugaya cohort that registered 1048 aged Japanese for 11 years. The primary outcome was the relationship between % FVC and mortality by cancer, cardiovascular disease, or pneumonia. Exposure variables were % FVC or leg force divided by 80% or median values, respectively. The secondary outcome was the effects of leg force on the relationship. Among the diseases, % FVC < 80% was related only to higher pneumonia mortality (hazard ratio [HR], 4.09; 95% CI, 1.90–8.83) relative to the % FVC ≥ 80% group before adjustment. Adding the leg force as an explanatory variable reduced the HR to 3.34 (1.54–7.25). Weak leg force might indicate sarcopenia, and its prevention may improve higher pneumonia mortality risk related to impaired % FVC, which we may advise people in clinical settings.

Keywords: forced vital capacity; muscle strength; older people; pneumonia mortality; sarcopenia; cohort study

Citation: Shiokawa, N.; Okazaki, T.; Suzukamo, Y.; Miyatake, M.; Kogure, M.; Nakaya, N.; Hozawa, A.; Ebihara, S.; Izumi, S.-I. Association between Low Forced Vital Capacity and High Pneumonia Mortality, and Impact of Muscle Power. *J. Clin. Med.* **2023**, *12*, 3272. https://doi.org/10.3390/jcm12093272

Academic Editor: Luca Quartuccio

Received: 31 March 2023
Revised: 27 April 2023
Accepted: 2 May 2023
Published: 4 May 2023

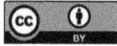

Copyright: © 2023 by the authors. Licensee MDPI, Basel, Switzerland. This article is an open access article distributed under the terms and conditions of the Creative Commons Attribution (CC BY) license (https:// creativecommons.org/licenses/by/ 4.0/).

1. Introduction

Major indicators of respiratory functions include forced vital capacity (FVC) and % predicted value FVC (% FVC). Previous studies showed that impaired FVC/% FVC were related to higher mortality in the general population [1–5]. In general, impaired FVC/% FVC are major indices for the diagnosis of interstitial lung disease, which is accompanied by higher mortality [6,7]. To exclude potential interstitial lung disease patients, two previous studies excluded people who complained about respiratory symptoms and showed that impaired FVC/% FVC were related to higher mortality [8,9].

Previous studies have reported that extremity muscle weakness was related to higher mortality [10–15]. There is a moderate correlation between the extremity and respiratory muscle strengths. In addition, there is a moderate correlation between FVC/% FVC and respiratory muscle power [16–19]. In aged adults, the development of pneumonia was related to respiratory muscle weakness [20]. Moreover, the possibility of a relationship between pneumonia-induced death and respiratory muscle weakness was suggested [20].

In aged males, strong leg force showed a potential to improve the relationship between impaired % FVC and higher mortality [9].

Currently, the disease that causes the relationship between higher mortality and impaired FVC/% FVC in the general population is unknown. Moreover, the effect of strong muscle force on the relationship between the disease-induced higher mortality and impaired FVC/% FVC is unknown.

The primary objective of this research was the identification of the disease that causes the relationship between higher mortality and impaired % FVC in aged adults. Next, this study aimed to identify the impact of strong leg force on the relationship between the disease-induced higher mortality and impaired % FVC.

The longitudinal cohort, the Tsurugaya project, was analyzed to identify the suggested objectives. We first evaluated a relationship between the impaired % FVC and the three major leading causes of death in Japan. The three major leading causes of death were cancer, cardiovascular disease, and pneumonia. We hypothesized the relationship between impaired % FVC and higher pneumonia mortality and the beneficial effects of the strong leg force on this relationship.

2. Materials and Methods

2.1. Participants

In 2002, the Tsurugaya project enrolled older adults aged ≥ 70 years and conducted comprehensive geriatric assessments [9]. The baseline data were collected by the survey performed in the assessments. We obtained informed consent from all participants involved in the study.

2.2. Examinations

We examined lung function using a spirometer (OST 80A, Chest Co., Tokyo, Japan). We took the best result among the 3 trials. We calculated the % FVC values based on participants' gender, age, and height [21]. We performed the first measurements in 2002 in accordance with the recommendation of the American Thoracic Society [22]. For the evaluation of FVC, we applied reference values announced by the Japanese Respiratory Society (JRS) in 2001. In addition, as a cut-off value for % FVC, we used 80%, announced by JRS in 2001. JRS announced the present reference values for Japanese in 2014; however, to be consistent with other Tsurugaya cohort studies, the reference values published in 2001 were applied in this study [23]. As for the leg force (w/kg), we evaluated its extension force using Combi Anaeropress3500 (Tokyo, Japan), a horizontal leg force measurement device [24]. The leg force was measured 5 times, and the average of the 2 strongest leg forces was calculated. We divided the average by the body weight [24]. We divided the participants into strong and weak leg force groups according to the median values of the gender-dependent leg force: ≥ 13.0 w/kg for males and ≥ 7.3 w/kg for females in the strong group. To evaluate dyspnea, we asked the participants to inspire through an external circuit. The external circuit was set with 3 steps of resistive load ($cmH_2O/L/s$); the lowest load was 10, the middle was 20, and the highest was 30. We asked them to report their feeling using the modified Borg scale. The modified Borg scale categorizes dyspnea on a scale from 0 to 10. The number 0 is scaled as no dyspnea, and the number 10 is the greatest dyspnea. As baseline breathing, the participants were asked to breathe without resistive load for 1 min. We excluded participants who selected 2 or greater at the baseline breathing as potential interstitial lung disease patients in the sensitivity analyses [9]. The questionnaire survey collected sociodemographic and medical information. Date of birth, gender, past medical history (pneumonia, malignant disease, heart disease, stroke, diabetes mellitus, and hypertension), smoking status, and medications with statins and angiotensin-converting enzyme (ACE) inhibitors were included in the questionnaire. We listed ACE inhibitors because they improve cough and swallowing reflexes and prevent the onset of pneumonia [25]. The smoking status was a categorical variable; we categorized the smoking status of participants into current, past, or never. We evaluated symptoms of depression using the Geriatric Depression Scale (GDS) written in Japanese with a 30-point scale [26], and examined cognitive function using the Mini–Mental State Examination (MMSE) written in Japanese [9]. Serum samples were isolated without asking for fasting, and a clinical testing laboratory assessed the serum albumin and total cholesterol concentrations.

2.3. Mortality Follow-Up

The primary endpoint was death from pneumonia, cancer, and cardiovascular disease. Causes of death were classified in accordance with the International Classification of Disease, 10th Revision (ICD10). Deaths from pneumonia were classified as J12–18 and 69; from cancer, deaths were classified as C0–26, 30–41, 43–58, 60–97; from cardiovascular diseases, deaths were classified as I20–28, 30–52, 60–89, and 95–99.

We obtained data regarding death from the Sendai Municipal Authority. We surveyed the cause of death by checking hospital records or the data submitted to the Japan arteriosclerosis longitudinal study coordinating center. The Japan arteriosclerosis longitudinal study involved 21 cohort studies in Japan and included the Tsurugaya project [27]. We followed the participants from 30 March 2003 to 1 July 2012.

2.4. Statistical Analysis

% FVC divided participants into 2 groups, and their characteristics at baseline were compared; chi-square tests compared categorical variables, and unpaired t-tests compared continuous variables. To evaluate the cumulative survival rate, we compared 2 groups divided by the % FVC. The Kaplan–Meier method and log-rank tests were used for the comparison. We calculated the hazard ratios (HRs) and 95% confidence intervals (CIs) of the mortality in this study using the Cox proportional hazard model. We set the reference group as the participants with % FVC $\geq$ 80%. Then, 2 models were ran to assess the correlation between the 2 groups for % FVC and mortality. Model 1 was defined as a model without adjustment. Gender and age were adjusted in Model 2. We also adjusted Model 2 with smoking. We divided the participants into 2 groups by the median values of the leg force. As the secondary outcome, we evaluated the impact of muscle force on the relationship between pneumonia mortality and % FVC divided into 2 groups. Model 1 was defined as a model without adjustment. In Model 2, we added leg force as an explanatory variable. Age and gender were adjusted in Model 3. Sensitivity analyses were performed for the evaluation of the robustness. The evaluated robustness was the relationship between mortality by pneumonia and % FVC divided into 2 groups. Statistical examinations were conducted using the software IBM SPSS Statistics 24.0 (International Business Machines Corporation, Armonk, NY, USA). We used the post hoc power analysis to evaluate the power of the main result. The software Power and Precision 4.1 (Biostat, Englewood, NJ, USA) was used for the evaluation. We interpreted $p < 0.05$ as statistically significant.

3. Results

In 2002, we recruited participants for the Tsurugaya project and invited all aged residents aged 70 years and older (n = 2730). At the baseline survey, 1198 participants were enrolled in the project. We obtained informed consent from 1175 participants. The study flow chart was shown in Figure 1. We excluded 19 participants without spirometry data. To keep the measured indices reliable, we used the Mini–Mental State Examination (MMSE). Participants missing the MMSE score or <10 were excluded (n = 8). Participants missing or with incomplete leg force measurement records were excluded (n = 80). Participants without serum laboratory data were also excluded (n = 20). Finally, we analyzed 1048 participants.

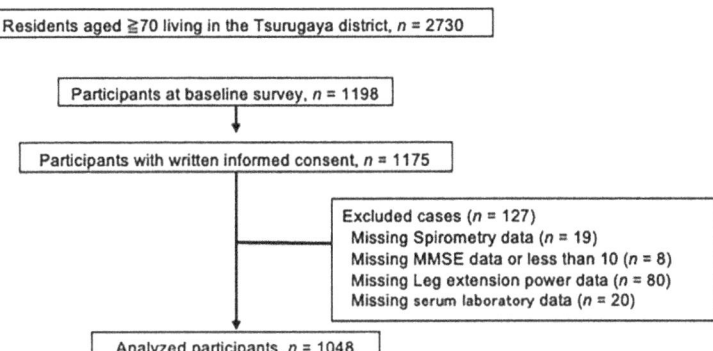

Figure 1. A schematic diagram outlining the enrollment in this study. MMSE = Mini–Mental State Examination.

To divide the participants into two groups by % FVC, we used its clinical cut-off value of 80%. The characteristics of the baseline survey are shown in Table 1. Males occupied 42.2% of the participants, and 75.7 (4.8) years of age, average (standard deviation [SD]), was the average age of the participants. Between the two groups, we found significant differences in gender, history of suffering from pneumonia, MMSE, current smoking status, leg extension force, total cholesterol level, and serum albumin level. However, the differences in the MMSE scores were small: 26.7 (3.4) in % FVC < 80% and 27.4 (2.6) in ≥80%. The albumin levels showed a similar trend: 4.34 (0.3) in % FVC < 80% and 4.30 (0.3) in ≥80%.

Table 1. The participants were divided by % FVC, and their baseline characteristics are shown.

Characteristics	Overall		% FVC <80%		% FVC ≥80%		p-Value *
Number of Participants	1048		223		825		
Age, mean (SD)	75.7	(4.8)	76.2	(4.5)	75.5	(4.9)	0.086
Men, n (%)	442	(42.2)	132	(59.2)	310	(37.6)	<0.001
Medical history, n (%)							
Pneumonia	100	(9.5)	35	(15.7)	65	(7.9)	<0.001
Cancer	70	(6.7)	12	(5.4)	58	(5.5)	0.451
Cardiovascular disease	161	(15.4)	34	(15.2)	127	(15.4)	0.957
Diabetes mellitus	146	(13.9)	36	(16.1)	110	(13.3)	0.278
Hypertension	392	(37.4)	92	(41.3)	300	(36.4)	0.180
Current smoking, n (%)	137	(13.4)	36	(16.4)	101	(12.5)	<0.001
MMSE, mean (SD)	27.3	(3.4)	26.7	(3.4)	27.4	(2.6)	0.048
Depressive symptoms, mean (SD)	9.0	(5.5)	9.3	(5.4)	8.9	(5.5)	0.356
Taking statins, n (%)	168	(16.0)	31	(13.9)	137	(16.6)	0.356
Taking ACE inhibitors, n (%)	78	(7.4)	17	(7.6)	61	(7.4)	0.886
Strong leg power †, n (%)	529	(50.5)	86	(38.6)	443	(53.7)	<0.001
Weak leg power ‡, n (%)	519	(49.5)	137	(61.4)	382	(46.3)	
Total cholesterol (mg/dL), mean (SD)	203.8	(33.3)	199.1	(35.7)	205.1	(32.6)	0.018
Albumin (g/dL), mean (SD)	4.3	(0.3)	4.34	(0.3)	4.30	(0.3)	0.043

% FVC = % predicted value forced vital capacity, SD = standard deviation, MMSE = Mini–Mental State Examination, ACE = angiotensin-converting enzyme, * Continuous variables were evaluated by unpaired t-test, and the chi-squared test evaluated proportion variables to obtain the data. † Strong leg power; leg extension force ≥13.0 w/kg (male), ≥7.3 w/kg (female). ‡ weak leg power; leg extension force <13.0 w/kg (male), <7.3 w/kg (female).

We previously showed the relationship between higher all-cause mortality and impaired % FVC in the Tsurugaya cohort [9]. Next, we determined the disease that caused the relationship between higher mortality and impaired FVC/% FVC among the three major leading causes of death in Japan. We analyzed the data registered in 2002 and followed until 2012. During the 8310 person years of follow-up, there were 57 deaths from cancer (251 person years), 38 deaths from cardiovascular diseases (180 person years), and 26 deaths from pneumonia (129 person years). We analyzed the relationship between mortality, and the % FVC was divided into ≥80% and <80% in each disease (Table 2). We set the reference group as the participants with % FVC ≥ 80%. Model 1 was defined as a model without adjustment. Gender and age were adjusted in Model 2. Among the pneumonia group, % FVC < 80% was related to higher mortality; the HR (95% CIs) was 4.09 (1.90 to 8.83) in Model 1 and 3.08 (1.41 to 6.71) in Model 2. In cancer and cardiovascular disease groups, % FVC < 80% was not related to higher mortality in either Model 1 or 2; the HRs were 1.08 (0.57 to 2.05) in cancer and 1.88 (0.95 to 3.74) in cardiovascular disease groups in Model 1. The adjustment for smoking in Model 2 did not essentially change the results; the HRs were 2.91 (1.33 to 6.33) in pneumonia, 0.87 (0.46 to 1.66) in cancer, and 1.57 (0.78 to 3.15) in cardiovascular disease groups. The power of the HRs of the pneumonia mortality was 0.97 with the total duration, hazard rates, and attrition rates; the sample size was 825 in the % FVC group ≥ 80%, and 223 in the % FVC group < 80%, and alpha (0.05, 1-tail).

Table 2. Relationship between % FVC divided into 2 groups and mortality by diseases.

	% FVC ≥ 80% (n = 825)	% FVC < 80% (n = 223)
Pneumonia death(n)	13	13
person years		129
Model 1	1.00 (Reference)	4.09 (1.90–8.83)
Model 2	1.00 (Reference)	3.08 (1.41–6.71)
Cancer death(n)	45	12
person years		251
Model 1	1.00 (Reference)	1.08 (0.57–2.05)
Model 2	1.00 (Reference)	0.87 (0.46–1.66)
CVD death(n)	26	12
person years		180
Model 1 [‡]	1.00 (Reference)	1.88 (0.95–3.74)
Model 2 [§]	1.00 (Reference)	1.61 (0.80–3.21)

Hazard ratio (95% confidence interval), % FVC = % predicted value forced vital capacity, [‡] Model 1: defined as a model without adjustment, [§] Model 2: sex and age were adjusted, CVD = cardiovascular diseases.

Next, sensitivity analyses of the relationship between % FVC and mortality were performed. Generally, interstitial lung disease patients are associated with higher mortality with impaired % FVC. Dyspnea is one of the typical symptoms of interstitial lung disease. Therefore, we evaluated dyspnea. Accordingly, we excluded 21 participants that had the potential to suffer from interstitial lung disease. The results did not essentially change after the exclusion; the HR was 3.75 (1.59 to 8.82) in Model 1 (Table A1). In general, aged pneumonia patients reach death by repeating the onset of pneumonia [17]. Thus, we excluded participants with a past history of pneumonia and conducted a sensitivity analysis. The results were somewhat confusing; the HR was 3.07 (1.31 to 7.18, $p = 0.010$) in Model 1 and 2.31 (0.98 to 5.45, $p = 0.056$) in Model 2 (Table A2).

The number of deaths caused by pneumonia was 13 (1.6%) out of the 825 participants in the % FVC ≥ 80% group and 13 (5.8%) out of the 223 participants in the % FVC < 80% group. Figure 2 shows Kaplan–Meier survival curves associated with death caused by pneumonia according to the FVC% predicted. The % FVC < 80% group showed a significantly lower cumulative survival rate than the % FVC ≥ 80% group (log-rank test, $p < 0.001$).

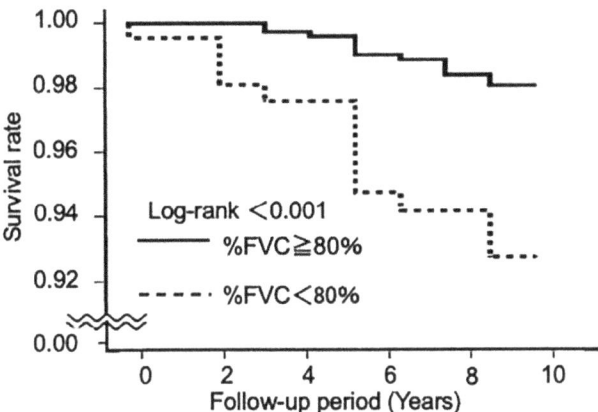

Figure 2. Kaplan–Meier survival curves showing the cumulative survival rates according to the FVC% predicted.

We next evaluated the impact of muscle force on the relationship between % FVC and pneumonia mortality. Model 1 was a univariate model of this relationship (Table 3). The participants were divided into two groups, strong and weak, by the gender-dependent median values of the leg force. We defined the reference group as the participants with % FVC ≥ 80% and a strong leg force group. We added the leg force as an explanatory variable to the % FVC in Model 1 and showed it in Model 2. In the % FVC < 80% group, we observed a reduction in the HR 3.34 (1.54 to 7.25) in Model 2, whereas it was 4.09 in Model 1. The leg force in Model 2, shown in Table 3, was an unadjusted model, and the weak leg force was related to higher mortality; the HR was 5.27 (1.81 to 15.41), which we interpreted as independent from % FVC. Model 3 was further adjusted for age and gender. The HR was 2.59 (1.18 to 5.68) for the % FVC < 80% group. An adjustment of Model 3 to smoking did not essentially change the results; the HR was 2.50 (1.14 to 5.47) for the % FVC < 80% group.

Table 3. The muscle force affected the relationship between mortality by pneumonia and % FVC divided by 80%.

	% FVC ≥ 80% Strong Leg Power ‡	% FVC < 80% Weak Leg Power §	p-Value
	Reference	HR (95% CI)	
Model 1			
FVC% predicted	1.00	4.09 (1.90–8.83)	<0.001
Model 2			
FVC% predicted	1.00	3.34 (1.54–7.25)	0.002
Leg power		5.27 (1.81–15.41)	0.003
Model 3			
FVC% predicted	1.00	2.59 (1.18–5.68)	0.017
Leg power		4.79 (1.59–14.45)	0.005

% FVC = % predicted value forced vital capacity, HR (95% CI) = hazard ratio (95% confidence interval), Model 1: defined as a model without adjustment, Model 2: leg power was split into 2 groups by the gender-dependent median values and added to Model 1, Model 3: sex and age were adjusted in Model 2, ‡ strong leg power; leg extension force ≥13.0 kg/w (male), ≥7.3 kg/w (female), § weak leg power; leg extension force <13.0 kg/w (male), <7.3 kg/w (female).

4. Discussion

Among the three major leading causes of death, impaired % FVC was related to higher pneumonia mortality in community-dwelling aged adults. Strong leg force may beneficially affect this relationship.

The follow-up period of this study was from 2003 to 2012. The four leading causes of death were cancer, heart disease, pneumonia, and cerebrovascular disease during this period in Japan. However, the number of deaths by cerebrovascular disease was 15, and was insufficient for analysis. Therefore, we gathered death by heart and cerebrovascular diseases and analyzed them as cardiovascular diseases. A previous study analyzed 1265 aged adults with chronic obstructive pulmonary disease, asthma, or other diseases and reported cause-specific mortality rates of % FVC < 80% [1]. They recruited participants between January 1996 to July 1999 and followed until 30 January 2002. They reported higher mortality rates with pulmonary and cerebrovascular diseases. In contrast to their study, our study did not recruit participants with specific diseases and carried out a long-term follow-up.

Respiratory function and extremity muscle strength have moderate correlations with respiratory muscle strength [16–19]. Respiratory muscle force regulates the effectiveness of coughing. The cough clears the airways and plays a central role in pneumonia protection [28]. Thus, strong leg force might beneficially affect the mortality risk of pneumonia via its correlation with respiratory muscle force and effective coughing.

Generally, sarcopenia is an aging-related muscle dysfunction defined by muscle weakness, low muscle mass, and performance [29]. Muscle weakness comes to the forefront among these indices [30]. A previous study showed that weak respiratory muscle force and low muscle mass were risk factors for the onset of pneumonia [20]. These data may link sarcopenia to the respiratory muscles. Sarcopenia is crucial because it is related to higher mortality [31,32]. This study showed that the impaired % FVC was related to higher pneumonia mortality with the possible involvement of the leg force. When we take the above links together, this study may support the following idea; sarcopenia in respiratory muscles causes respiratory-related diseases, such as pneumonia, due to ineffective coughing and is possibly connected to death.

Interstitial lung disease patients show impaired % FVC and higher mortality [6]. Their common respiratory symptoms are dyspnea and coughing. This study examined dyspnea and attempted to exclude the participants that had the potential to suffer from interstitial lung disease. However, they might not have symptoms or impaired pulmonary functions. Thus, it is difficult to entirely exclude the participants with the potential to suffer from interstitial lung disease in the sensitivity analysis. The prevalence of interstitial lung disease patients was reported as approximately 6.3–76.0 cases per 100,000 people [7]. This study excluded 21 participants among 1048. Therefore, in addition to interstitial lung disease patients, non-interstitial lung disease patients might be excluded from the sensitivity analysis.

We previously reported the beneficial effect of the strong leg force on the relationship between all-cause mortality and impaired % FVC in males but not in females [9]. Since pneumonia caused only six deaths in females in this study, we could not divide the participants by gender for further analysis. However, the strong leg force improved the relationship after adjustment for gender. Thus, other diseases than pneumonia might cause gender-dependent beneficial effects of the strong leg force on the relationship, or this may be a limitation of the current study. In addition, from the point of view of medical care costs, the costs were inversely associated with physical activity in aged adults [24]. The strength of the leg force partially represents physical activity [24]. Thus, strengthening the leg force and improving physical activity might have the potential of preventing pneumonia in addition to reducing medical care costs.

This study has some limitations. First, the participants were Japanese/East Asians, and the ethnicity of the sample was limited. Therefore, we may apply our results to Asian populations, but not to other ethnicities. Second, the number of pneumonia deaths was insufficient for numerous-factor adjustments. Third, we could not analyze data on the immune system, which plays essential roles in multiple diseases, especially in infectious diseases such as pneumonia [25,33,34]. Fourth, after excluding the past history of pneumonia in the sensitivity analysis, we encountered difficulties in the interpretation of the discrepancy of the HRs between Models 1 and 2. One possible explanation was that we could not know when the pneumonia developed, i.e., in youth or old age.

This study characterized the specific disease as pneumonia, which causes the relationship between impaired % FVC and higher mortality in community-dwelling aged adults. Preventing weak leg force may reduce mortality risk. Since we currently have few management strategies to improve FVC, we may suggest the potential benefits of strengthening muscle force to community-dwelling aged adults with impaired % FVC.

Author Contributions: N.S.: Methodology, analysis, and writing. T.O.: Conceptualization, investigation, and writing. Y.S.: Methodology, analysis, and writing. M.M.: Methodology and analysis. M.K.: Data curation, project administration, and resources. N.N.: Data curation, project administration, resources, and investigation. A.H. and S.E.: Data curation, project administration, resources, investigation, and writing. S.-I.I.: Conceptualization and supervision. All authors have read and agreed to the published version of the manuscript.

Funding: This study was supported by a Grant-In-Aid for Scientific Research from the Japan Society for the Promotion of the Science to T.O. (18K08133 and 22H029643), by AMED to T.O. (under grant number 17dk0110024 and no. 19dk0310101h0001), and by The General Insurance Association of Japan to T.O.

Institutional Review Board Statement: This study was conducted in accordance with the guidelines of the Declaration of Helsinki, and approved by the Ethics Committee of Tohoku University Graduate School of Medicine (approval number: 2002040).

Informed Consent Statement: Informed consent was obtained from all participants involved in the study.

Data Availability Statement: The data that support the findings of this study are available from A.H. upon reasonable request.

Conflicts of Interest: The authors declare no conflict of interest.

Appendix A

Table A1. The association between % FVC and pneumonia mortality after excluding potential interstitial lung disease patients.

	% FVC ≥ 80%	% FVC < 80%	p-Value
	Reference	HR (95%CI)	
Model 1	1.00	3.75 (1.59–8.82)	0.003
Model 2	1.00	2.93 (1.23–6.98)	0.016

% FVC = % predicted value forced vital capacity, HR (95% CI) = hazard ratio (95% confidence interval), Model 1: defined as a model without adjustment, Model 2: sex and age were adjusted.

Table A2. The relationship between % FVC and pneumonia mortality after the exclusion of participants with a past history of pneumonia.

	% FVC ≥ 80%	% FVC < 80%	p-Value
	Reference	HR (95%CI)	
Model 1	1.00	3.07 (1.31–7.18)	0.010
Model 2	1.00	2.31 (0.98–5.45)	0.056

%FVC = % predicted value forced vital capacity, HR (95% CI) = hazard ratio (95% confidence interval), Model 1: defined as a model without adjustment, Model 2: sex and age were adjusted.

References

1. Scarlata, S.; Pedone, C.; Fimognari, F.L.; Bellia, V.; Forastiere, F.; Incalzi, R.A. Restrictive pulmonary dysfunction at spirometry and mortality in the elderly. *Respir. Med.* **2008**, *102*, 1349–1354. [CrossRef]
2. Magnussen, C.; Ojeda, F.M.; Rzayeva, N.; Zeller, T.; Sinning, C.R.; Pfeiffer, N.; Beutel, M.; Blettner, M.; Lackner, K.J.; Blankenberg, S.; et al. FEV1 and FVC predict all-cause mortality independent of cardiac function—Results from the population-based Gutenberg Health Study. *Int. J. Cardiol.* **2017**, *234*, 64–68. [CrossRef]

3. Breet, Y.; Schutte, A.E.; Huisman, H.W.; Eloff, F.C.; Du Plessis, J.L.; Kruger, A.; Van Rooyen, J.M. Lung function, inflammation and cardiovascular mortality in Africans. *Eur. J. Clin. Investig.* **2016**, *46*, 901–910. [CrossRef]
4. Mannino, D.M.; Buist, A.S.; Petty, T.L.; Enright, P.L.; Redd, S.C. Lung function and mortality in the United States: Data from the First National Health and Nutrition Examination Survey follow up study. *Thorax* **2003**, *58*, 388–393. [CrossRef]
5. Vaz Fragoso, C.A.; Van Ness, P.H.; Murphy, T.E.; McAvay, G.J. Spirometric impairments, cardiovascular outcomes, and noncardiovascular death in older persons. *Respir. Med.* **2018**, *137*, 40–47. [CrossRef]
6. Putman, R.K.; Hatabu, H.; Araki, T.; Gudmundsson, G.; Gao, W.; Nishino, M.; Okajima, Y.; Dupuis, J.; Latourelle, J.C.; Cho, M.H.; et al. Association Between Interstitial Lung Abnormalities and All-Cause Mortality. *JAMA* **2016**, *315*, 672–681. [CrossRef]
7. Wijsenbeek, M.; Suzuki, A.; Maher, T.M. Interstitial lung diseases. *Lancet* **2022**, *400*, 769–786. [CrossRef]
8. Burney, P.G.; Hooper, R. Forced vital capacity, airway obstruction and survival in a general population sample from the USA. *Thorax* **2011**, *66*, 49–54. [CrossRef]
9. Miyatake, M.; Okazaki, T.; Suzukamo, Y.; Matsuyama, S.; Tsuji, I.; Izumi, S.I. High Mortality in an Older Japanese Population with Low Forced Vital Capacity and Gender-Dependent Potential Impact of Muscle Strength: Longitudinal Cohort Study. *J. Clin. Med.* **2022**, *11*, 5264. [CrossRef]
10. Laukkanen, P.; Heikkinen, E.; Kauppinen, M. Muscle strength and mobility as predictors of survival in 75-84-year-old people. *Age Ageing* **1995**, *24*, 468–473. [CrossRef]
11. Metter, E.J.; Talbot, L.A.; Schrager, M.; Conwit, R. Skeletal muscle strength as a predictor of all-cause mortality in healthy men. *J. Gerontol. A Biol. Sci. Med. Sci.* **2002**, *57*, B359–B365. [CrossRef]
12. Takata, Y.; Shimada, M.; Ansai, T.; Yoshitake, Y.; Nishimuta, M.; Nakagawa, N.; Ohashi, M.; Yoshihara, A.; Miyazaki, H. Physical performance and 10-year mortality in a 70-year-old community-dwelling population. *Aging Clin. Exp. Res.* **2012**, *24*, 257–264. [CrossRef]
13. Celis-Morales, C.A.; Welsh, P.; Lyall, D.M.; Steell, L.; Petermann, F.; Anderson, J.; Iliodromiti, S.; Sillars, A.; Graham, N.; Mackay, D.F.; et al. Associations of grip strength with cardiovascular, respiratory, and cancer outcomes and all cause mortality: Prospective cohort study of half a million UK Biobank participants. *BMJ* **2018**, *361*, k1651. [CrossRef]
14. Newman, A.B.; Kupelian, V.; Visser, M.; Simonsick, E.M.; Goodpaster, B.H.; Kritchevsky, S.B.; Tylavsky, F.A.; Rubin, S.M.; Harris, T.B. Strength, but not muscle mass, is associated with mortality in the health, aging and body composition study cohort. *J. Gerontol. A Biol. Sci. Med. Sci.* **2006**, *61*, 72–77. [CrossRef]
15. Gale, C.R.; Martyn, C.N.; Cooper, C.; Sayer, A.A. Grip strength, body composition, and mortality. *Int. J. Epidemiol.* **2007**, *36*, 228–235. [CrossRef]
16. Enright, P.L.; Kronmal, R.A.; Manolio, T.A.; Schenker, M.B.; Hyatt, R.E. Respiratory muscle strength in the elderly. Correlates and reference values. Cardiovascular Health Study Research Group. *Am. J. Respir. Crit. Care Med.* **1994**, *149*, 430–438. [CrossRef]
17. Okazaki, T.; Ebihara, S.; Mori, T.; Izumi, S.; Ebihara, T. Association between sarcopenia and pneumonia in older people. *Geriatr. Gerontol. Int.* **2020**, *20*, 7–13. [CrossRef]
18. Shin, H.I.; Kim, D.K.; Seo, K.M.; Kang, S.H.; Lee, S.Y.; Son, S. Relation Between Respiratory Muscle Strength and Skeletal Muscle Mass and Hand Grip Strength in the Healthy Elderly. *Ann. Rehabil. Med.* **2017**, *41*, 686–692. [CrossRef]
19. Buchman, A.S.; Boyle, P.A.; Wilson, R.S.; Gu, L.; Bienias, J.L.; Bennett, D.A. Pulmonary function, muscle strength and mortality in old age. *Mech. Ageing Dev.* **2008**, *129*, 625–631. [CrossRef]
20. Okazaki, T.; Suzukamo, Y.; Miyatake, M.; Komatsu, R.; Yaekashiwa, M.; Nihei, M.; Izumi, S.; Ebihara, T. Respiratory Muscle Weakness as a Risk Factor for Pneumonia in Older People. *Gerontology* **2021**, *67*, 581–590. [CrossRef]
21. Kubota, M.; Kobayashi, H.; Quanjer, P.H.; Omori, H.; Tatsumi, K.; Kanazawa, M.; Clinical Pulmonary Functions Committee of the Japanese Respiratory Society. Reference values for spirometry, including vital capacity, in Japanese adults calculated with the LMS method and compared with previous values. *Respir. Investig.* **2014**, *52*, 242–250. [CrossRef]
22. Standardization of Spirometry, 1994 Update. American Thoracic Society. *Am. J. Respir. Crit. Care Med.* **1995**, *152*, 1107–1136. [CrossRef]
23. Ebihara, S.; Niu, K.; Ebihara, T.; Kuriyama, S.; Hozawa, A.; Ohmori-Matsuda, K.; Nakaya, N.; Nagatomi, R.; Arai, H.; Kohzuki, M.; et al. Impact of blunted perception of dyspnea on medical care use and expenditure, and mortality in elderly people. *Front. Physiol.* **2012**, *3*, 238. [CrossRef]
24. Yang, G.; Niu, K.; Fujita, K.; Hozawa, A.; Ohmori-Matsuda, K.; Kuriyama, S.; Nakaya, N.; Ebihara, S.; Okazaki, T.; Guo, H.; et al. Impact of physical activity and performance on medical care costs among the Japanese elderly. *Geriatr. Gerontol. Int.* **2011**, *11*, 157–165. [CrossRef]
25. Nihei, M.; Okazaki, T.; Ebihara, S.; Kobayashi, M.; Niu, K.; Gui, P.; Tamai, T.; Nukiwa, T.; Yamaya, M.; Kikuchi, T.; et al. Chronic inflammation, lymphangiogenesis, and effect of an anti-VEGFR therapy in a mouse model and in human patients with aspiration pneumonia. *J. Pathol.* **2015**, *235*, 632–645. [CrossRef]
26. Kuriyama, S.; Koizumi, Y.; Matsuda-Ohmori, K.; Seki, T.; Shimazu, T.; Hozawa, A.; Awata, S.; Tsuji, I. Obesity and depressive symptoms in elderly Japanese: The Tsurugaya Project. *J. Psychosom. Res.* **2006**, *60*, 229–235. [CrossRef]
27. Japan Arteriosclerosis Longitudinal Study, G. Japan Arteriosclerosis Longitudinal Study-Existing Cohorts Combine (JALS-ECC): Rationale, design, and population characteristics. *Circ. J.* **2008**, *72*, 1563–1568. [CrossRef]

28. Komatsu, R.; Okazaki, T.; Ebihara, S.; Kobayashi, M.; Tsukita, Y.; Nihei, M.; Sugiura, H.; Niu, K.; Ebihara, T.; Ichinose, M. Aspiration pneumonia induces muscle atrophy in the respiratory, skeletal, and swallowing systems. *J. Cachexia Sarcopenia Muscle* **2018**, *9*, 643–653. [CrossRef]
29. Cruz-Jentoft, A.J.; Bahat, G.; Bauer, J.; Boirie, Y.; Bruyere, O.; Cederholm, T.; Cooper, C.; Landi, F.; Rolland, Y.; Sayer, A.A.; et al. Sarcopenia: Revised European consensus on definition and diagnosis. *Age Ageing* **2019**, *48*, 601. [CrossRef]
30. Bhasin, S.; Travison, T.G.; Manini, T.M.; Patel, S.; Pencina, K.M.; Fielding, R.A.; Magaziner, J.M.; Newman, A.B.; Kiel, D.P.; Cooper, C.; et al. Sarcopenia Definition: The Position Statements of the Sarcopenia Definition and Outcomes Consortium. *J. Am. Geriatr. Soc.* **2020**, *68*, 1410–1418. [CrossRef]
31. Chen, L.K.; Woo, J.; Assantachai, P.; Auyeung, T.W.; Chou, M.Y.; Iijima, K.; Jang, H.C.; Kang, L.; Kim, M.; Kim, S.; et al. Asian Working Group for Sarcopenia: 2019 Consensus Update on Sarcopenia Diagnosis and Treatment. *J. Am. Med. Di.r Assoc.* **2020**, *21*, 300–307.e2. [CrossRef] [PubMed]
32. Guo, Y.; Niu, K.; Okazaki, T.; Wu, H.; Yoshikawa, T.; Ohrui, T.; Furukawa, K.; Ichinose, M.; Yanai, K.; Arai, H.; et al. Coffee treatment prevents the progression of sarcopenia in aged mice in vivo and in vitro. *Exp. Gerontol.* **2014**, *50*, 1–8. [CrossRef] [PubMed]
33. Tsukita, Y.; Okazaki, T.; Ebihara, S.; Komatsu, R.; Nihei, M.; Kobayashi, M.; Hirano, T.; Sugiura, H.; Tamada, T.; Tanaka, N.; et al. Beneficial effects of sunitinib on tumor microenvironment and immunotherapy targeting death receptor5. *Oncoimmunology* **2019**, *8*, e1543526. [CrossRef] [PubMed]
34. Ngamsnae, P.; Okazaki, T.; Ren, Y.; Xia, Y.; Hashimoto, H.; Ikeda, R.; Honkura, Y.; Katori, Y.; Izumi, S.I. Anatomy and pathology of lymphatic vessels under physiological and inflammatory conditions in the mouse diaphragm. *Microvasc. Res.* **2023**, *145*, 104438. [CrossRef]

Disclaimer/Publisher's Note: The statements, opinions and data contained in all publications are solely those of the individual author(s) and contributor(s) and not of MDPI and/or the editor(s). MDPI and/or the editor(s) disclaim responsibility for any injury to people or property resulting from any ideas, methods, instructions or products referred to in the content.

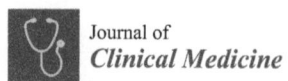

Systematic Review

The Clinical Significance of Anaerobic Coverage in the Antibiotic Treatment of Aspiration Pneumonia: A Systematic Review and Meta-Analysis

Yuki Yoshimatsu [1,2], Masaharu Aga [3], Kosaku Komiya [4,*], Shusaku Haranaga [5], Yuka Numata [6], Makoto Miki [7], Futoshi Higa [8], Kazuyoshi Senda [9] and Shinji Teramoto [10]

1. Elderly Care, Queen Elizabeth Hospital, Lewisham and Greenwich NHS Trust, London SE18 4QH, UK
2. Centre for Exercise Activity and Rehabilitation, School of Human Sciences, University of Greenwich, London SE9 2HB, UK
3. Department of Respiratory Medicine, Yokohama Municipal Citizen's Hospital, Yokohama 221-0855, Japan
4. Respiratory Medicine and Infectious Diseases, Oita University Faculty of Medicine, Yufu 879-5593, Japan
5. Comprehensive Health Professions Education Center, University Hospital, University of the Ryukyus, Okinawa 903-0125, Japan
6. Department of Respiratory Medicine, Nagaoka Red Cross Hospital, Nagaoka 940-2085, Japan
7. Department of Respiratory Medicine, Japanese Red Cross Sendai Hospital, Sendai 982-0801, Japan
8. Department of Respiratory Medicine, National Hospital Organization Okinawa National Hospital, Okinawa 901-2214, Japan
9. Department Pharmacy, Kinjo Gakuin University, Nagoya 463-8521, Japan
10. Department of Respiratory Medicine, Tokyo Medical University Hachioji Medical Center, Tokyo 160-0023, Japan
* Correspondence: komiyakh1@oita-u.ac.jp; Tel.: +81-97-586-5110

Abstract: Introduction: Aspiration pneumonia is increasingly recognised as a common condition. While antibiotics covering anaerobes are thought to be necessary based on old studies reporting anaerobes as causative organisms, recent studies suggest that it may not necessarily benefit prognosis, or even be harmful. Clinical practice should be based on current data reflecting the shift in causative bacteria. The aim of this review was to investigate whether anaerobic coverage is recommended in the treatment of aspiration pneumonia. Methods: A systematic review and meta-analysis of studies comparing antibiotics with and without anaerobic coverage in the treatment of aspiration pneumonia was performed. The main outcome studied was mortality. Additional outcomes were resolution of pneumonia, development of resistant bacteria, length of stay, recurrence, and adverse effects. The Preferred Reporting Items for Systematic reviews and Meta-Analyses (PRISMA) guidelines were followed. Results: From an initial 2523 publications, one randomised control trial and two observational studies were selected. The studies did not show a clear benefit of anaerobic coverage. Upon meta-analysis, there was no benefit of anaerobic coverage in improving mortality (Odds ratio 1.23, 95% CI 0.67–2.25). Studies reporting resolution of pneumonia, length of hospital stay, recurrence of pneumonia, and adverse effects showed no benefit of anaerobic coverage. The development of resistant bacteria was not discussed in these studies. Conclusion: In the current review, there are insufficient data to assess the necessity of anaerobic coverage in the antibiotic treatment of aspiration pneumonia. Further studies are needed to determine which cases require anaerobic coverage, if any.

Keywords: dysphagia; swallowing impairment; pneumonia; anaerobe; anaerobic coverage; antibiotic; treatment

1. Introduction

Aspiration pneumonia has become a leading cause of hospitalisation and death in adults. It represents a major socioeconomic burden worldwide, accounting for up to 90% of pneumonia in the older population [1]. Within community-acquired and hospital-acquired pneumonia, aspiration pneumonia is a subtype known to have a poor prognosis [2]. Therefore, it is crucial to investigate the current optimal management of aspiration pneumonia.

Anaerobic bacteria have been thought to play a major role in the pathogenesis of aspiration pneumonia. This was particularly true in the 1970s [3–7], when several reports identified anaerobes as the causative organisms, and new antibiotics were developed to treat them. As a result of these findings, it became common practice to consider routine anaerobic coverage in patients suspected of having aspiration pneumonia [8].

However, recent studies suggest that anaerobic coverage may not necessarily improve clinical outcomes. A shift in the bacteria commonly associated with community-acquired pneumonia (CAP) and hospital-acquired pneumonia (HAP) has been reported, with fewer anaerobes identified [3,8,9]. Recent guidelines have taken these findings into account and do not recommend the routine coverage of anaerobic pathogens in the treatment of aspiration pneumonia [10,11].

As a result of these changes, it cannot be assumed that the optimal routine antibiotic treatment for aspiration pneumonia is to cover anaerobes. There is evidence that the routine usage of anaerobic coverage may not only be non-beneficial, but also potentially harmful [12,13]. The unnecessary use of broad-spectrum antibiotics must be avoided in view of future resistance, adverse effects and healthcare costs.

There have been review articles on aspiration pneumonia, providing overviews on their pathology and management [9,14,15]. These reviews have all commented on the shift in the role of anaerobes in aspiration pneumonia over the years, and questioned the routine usage of antibiotics that cover anaerobic organisms. However, to our knowledge, no formal systematic review has been published comparing clinical outcomes with or without anaerobic coverage in the treatment of aspiration pneumonia. Clinical practice and guideline updates should reflect the most recent evidence available. Therefore, we performed a systematic review of the literature to answer the question: "Is anaerobic coverage recommended in the treatment of aspiration pneumonia?".

2. Materials and Methods

A systematic review and meta-analysis of the scientific literature on the clinical significance of antibiotics with anaerobic coverage compared to antibiotics without anaerobic coverage in the treatment of aspiration pneumonia was performed. The Preferred Reporting Items for Systematic reviews and Meta-Analyses (PRISMA) guidelines were followed [16]. The protocol was registered to Prospero before initiation of the study (registration number: CRD42022358664) and can be found at the following URL: https://www.crd.york.ac.uk/prospero/display_record.php?RecordID=358664, accessed on 15 September 2022.

Patients were adults aged 18 years or older with a diagnosis of aspiration pneumonia, necrotising pneumonia or lung abscess. We added necrotising pneumonia and lung abscess so we do not exclude any potentially relevant studies, as aspiration pneumonia is still a variable term. The intervention was antimicrobial treatment covering anaerobic organisms. The control was antimicrobial treatment without coverage of anaerobic organisms. The main outcome studied was mortality, and other outcomes consisted of resolution of pneumonia, development of resistant bacteria, length of hospital stay, recurrence of pneumonia, and adverse effects. The types of studies included were primary studies published in a peer-reviewed journal. Studies from any setting and any year were included. All non-English literature, unpublished material, study protocols, conference abstracts, and book chapters were excluded to maintain the scientific quality of the review. Reviews were also excluded as they are not primary studies.

The databases searched were PubMed (https://pubmed.ncbi.nlm.nih.gov/, accessed on 15 September 2022) and Cochrane Library (https://www.cochranelibrary.com/, accessed on 15 September 2022). The search strategy was developed in PubMed and then subsequently translated for the Cochrane Library. Full strategies are provided in the Appendices A.1 and A.2. We searched for 'aspiration pneumonia' and 'treatment' using both controlled vocabulary, such as MeSH terms, and natural language terms for their synonyms. The search strategy was developed with broad terms to ensure all relevant articles would be detected in the database search. We excluded guidelines, meta-analyses, reviews, and case reports. The search was conducted on 7 September 2022. Duplicates were removed before screening using Rayyan duplicate identification strategies.

Identified studies were independently reviewed by two of the authors (Y.Y. and M.A.), and decisions were recorded using Rayyan. Disagreements were resolved by discussion and, where necessary, by review by two other authors (S.H. and Y.N.).

Inclusion criteria were original papers comparing antibacterial treatment with and without anaerobic coverage in adults (aged 18 years and older) diagnosed with aspiration pneumonia, necrotising pneumonia, or lung abscess. Exclusion criteria were reviews, case reports, editorials, conference papers, children, animals, in vitro studies, prophylactic antibiotics, and non-systemic routes of administration. Reviews were excluded from the study, but their references were searched for relevant studies. Manual searches of the reference lists of relevant guidelines [10,11,17], included studies, and other relevant publications [9,18,19] were also performed.

A data extraction form was designed to extract study characteristics and outcomes. Two reviewers (Y.Y. and M.A.) independently extracted data from eligible publications independently. The extracted data were compared, and any discrepancies were resolved by discussion between them and two other reviewers (S.H. and Y.N.). No automated tools were used. Data (odds ratio) on the primary outcome (mortality) and secondary outcomes (clinical cure rate, development of resistant bacteria, length of hospital stay, recurrence of pneumonia, and rate of adverse effects) were extracted. We also extracted information on the characteristics of the eligible studies and outcomes as follows: author, year, source of publication, sample size, sample/participant characteristics. If necessary, the authors of the publications were contacted.

Meta-analysis was performed using ReviewManager (Revman) (London, UK) for outcomes for which two or more studies provided data. For other outcomes for which only one study provided data, extracted data are presented and summarised descriptively.

The risk of bias of the observational studies [20,21] was assessed using the Newcastle Ottawa Scale (NOS) [22]. The NOS was also used to assess the randomised control trial (RCT) [23] for outcomes reported in two or more studies (mortality and clinical cure rate), to ensure consistency within outcomes. The Cohort Studies version of the scale was chosen to assess studies for subject selection, cohort comparability, and outcomes. The Cochrane Risk of Bias tool (RoB 2) was used for outcomes where only RCTs were included [24]. Two reviewers (Y.Y. and S.A.) independently assessed the risk of bias for each study, and any discrepancies were resolved by discussion.

3. Results

A total of 2728 studies were identified through database and manual searches. After removing 205 duplicates, 2523 reports were screened on their titles and abstracts, of which 2519 were excluded (Figure 1). The reasons for exclusion at the screening stage were: wrong population ($n = 1437$), wrong publication type ($n = 407$), wrong intervention ($n = 176$), background article ($n = 168$), wrong study design ($n = 147$), wrong language ($n = 144$), and wrong outcome ($n = 40$). Of the four studies that underwent full-text review, one was excluded due to incorrect study design [25]. Finally, three papers were included in the final analysis [20,21,23]. The study selection process is shown in Figure 1, according to the PRISMA methodology [16].

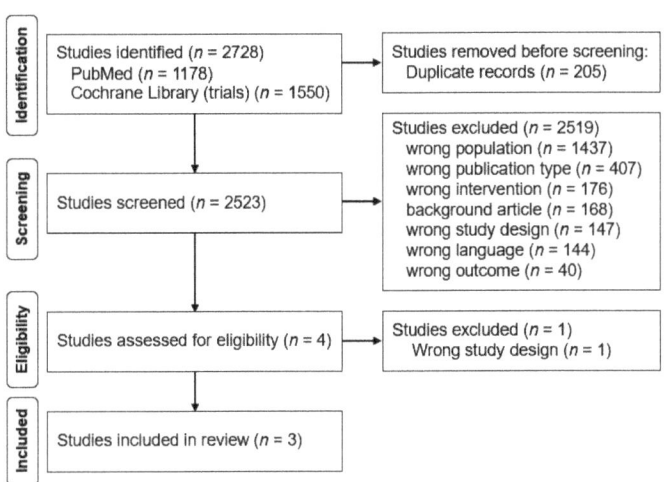

Figure 1. Flow chart of the study process. Through searching databases, 2728 reports were found. After removing duplicates, 2523 reports were screened, of which 2519 were excluded. A total of four studies underwent full-text review, and three studies were included in the review.

Of the three included studies, one was an RCT [23], and two were prospective observational studies [20,21]. A total of 941 subjects were included. All studies were conducted in Japan. All included studies had a mean/median age over 77 years. Their diagnoses were pneumonia with aspiration-related risk factors [21,23], or aspiration pneumonia within the NHCAP group B [20]. There was no mention of necrotising pneumonia or lung abscesses in the three studies. The characteristics of the studies are shown in Table 1. The propensity score-matched data by Hasegawa, et al. [21] were further analysed with multiple imputation by employed chain equations, and the data were not presented as integers. Therefore, raw data were used for meta-analysis to match the data in the two other studies.

Table 1. Study Characteristics.

Author, Year	Country	Design	Setting	Subjects	Age (Years)	Antibiotics (Number of Subjects)	
						Anaerobic Coverage Group	Control Group
Oi, 2022 [23]	Japan	Open-labeled Randomized comparative trial	Single centre, inpatient	Moderate to severe CAP/NHCAP patients at risk of aspiration	mean 85	MEPM (86)	CFPM (101)
Hasegawa, 2019 [21]	Japan	Prospective observational	Multicentre, inpatient/outpatient	Pneumonia patients with aspiration-related risk factor	median 77	SBT/ABPC (400)	CTRX (237)
Marumo, 2014 [20]	Japan	Prospective observational	Single centre, inpatient/outpatient	Aspiration pneumonia within the NHCAP group B (no risk of MDR pathogen)	mean 78	SBT/ABPC (81)	AZM (36)

CAP: community acquired pneumonia; NHCAP: nursing-and healthcare-associated pneumonia; MEPM: meropenem; CFPM: cefepime; SBT/ABPC: sulbactam/ampicillin; AZM: azithromycin.

Results for mortality and clinical cure rates are shown in Table 2 and Figure 2. The primary outcome and mortality were reported in all 3 studies; Oi et al. [23] reported 30-day mortality, whereas Hasegawa et al. [21] and Marumo et al. [20] reported in-hospital mortality. Overall, mortality was low and there was no significant mortality benefit in the anaerobic coverage group compared with the control group. Mortality was 9.9% (56/567) in the anaerobic coverage group, and 8.0% (30/374) in the control group (odds ratio (OR) 1.24, 95% confidence interval (CI) 0.70, 2.18).

Table 2. Mortality and clinical cure rate.

Author, Year	Mortality (30 Day * or in Hospital)			Clinical Cure Rate (n, %)		
	Anaerobic Coverage	Control	OR, 95%CI	Anaerobic Coverage	Control	OR, 95%CI
Oi, 2020 [23]	7/86 * (8.1%)	12/101 * (11.9%)	0.66 [0.25, 1.75]	73/86 (84.9%)	83/101 (82.2%)	1.22 [0.56, 2.66]
Hasegawa, 2019 [21]	40/400 (10.0%)	15/237 (6.3%)	1.64 [0.89, 3.05]	NR	NR	NR
Marumo, 2014 [20]	9/81 (11.1%)	3/36 (8.3%)	1.38 [0.35, 5.41]	60/81 (74.1%)	24/36 (66.7%)	1.43 [0.61, 3.35]

OR: odds ratio, CI: confidence interval, NR: not reported.

A

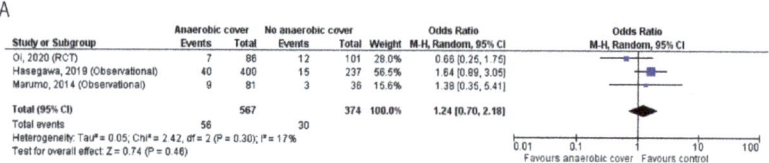

B

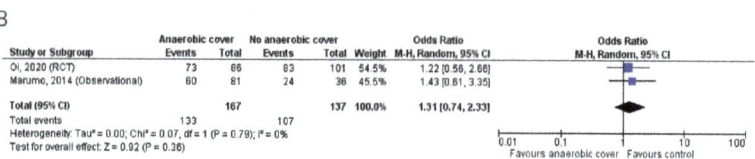

Figure 2. (A) Mortality; (B) Clinical cure rate. Forest plots comparing outcomes in groups given antibiotic treatment with or without anaerobic coverage. The blue square represents the odds ratios of individual studies. The black diamond represents the pooled result [20,21,23].

The clinical cure rate from two studies [20,23] showed no significant benefit of anaerobic coverage; the results were 79.6% (133/167) for the anaerobic coverage group, and 78.1% (107/137) for the control group, using the intention to treat analysis (OR 1.31, 95% CI 0.74, 2.33).

Length of hospital stay was reported in only one study [20]; 22.3 ± 7.3 days in the anaerobic coverage group, and 20.5 ± 8.1 days in the control group, with no significant difference ($p = 0.654$). Hasegawa et al. [21] reported the '28-day hospital-free days' as a substitute for length of stay, which was significantly shorter in the anaerobic coverage group than in the control group (11 vs. 9 days; $p = 0.005$).

The rate of pneumonia recurrence was reported in one RCT [23], and it was 5.8% (5/86) in the anaerobic coverage group, and 2.0% (2/101) in the control group, using the intention to treat analysis (OR 1.97, 95% CI 0.46, 8.48).

The rate of adverse effects was also reported in one RCT [23] only, in which the rate was 22.0% (18/82) in the anaerobic coverage group, and 25.5% (24/94) in the control group, using the validated per-protocol analysis (OR 0.82, 95% CI 0.41, 1.65). No serious antibiotic-related events were reported.

The rate of development of resistant bacteria was not reported in any of the three studies.

The risk of bias assessment using the NOS is shown in Table 3. All studies were rated low in the representativeness of the expressed cohort, as they had variable definitions of aspiration pneumonia and were limited to certain severity groups. Otherwise, they were generally graded well for most of the criteria for subject selection, cohort comparability, and outcome. For the outcomes for which only one RCT was included (recurrence rate and adverse effects), the risk of bias was assessed as 'low risk' using the RoB 2. However, as all studies were conducted in the acute setting in Japan, with mostly inpatients, this raises a concern regarding external validity. Therefore, it can be concluded that although there are issues with external validity, the risk of bias and internal validity is generally acceptable.

Table 3. Risk of bias assessment, Newcastle–Ottawa Scale.

	Selection				Comparability	Outcome			
Author, Year	Representativeness of Exposed Cohort	Selection of Controls	Ascertainment of Exposure	Demonstration that Outcome of Interest Was Not Present at Start of Study	Comparability of Cohorts on the Basis of the Design or Analysis	Assessment of Outcome	Adequate Length of Follow-up	Adequacy of Follow up of Cohorts	Total Score
Oi, 2020 [23]	b	a	a	a	a	c	a	a	7
Hasegawa, 2019 [21]	b	a	a	a	a	c	a	a	7
Marumo, 2014 [20]	c	a	a	a	a	c	a	a	6

(a, b, and c were allotted according to the criteria as defined by the Newcastle-Ottawa Scale [22]).

A funnel plot was generated to assess reporting bias (Appendix A.3, Figure A1). There appeared to be funnel plot symmetry for in-hospital mortality, although Sterne's test was not appropriate to detect funnel plot asymmetry due to the small number of studies included in each meta-analysis.

The overall certainty of evidence and the reasons for lowering the ratings are summarised in Table 4. The certainty of evidence was generally low or very low due to the limited availability of RCTs.

Table 4. Summary of findings.

Outcomes	No of Participants (Studies)	Odds Ratio [95% CI]	Certainty of Evidence (GRADE)	Reason for GRADing	Comments
Mortality	941 (3)	1.24 [0.70, 2.18]	Very low	Risk of bias, imprecision	There may be little or no difference in the mortality.
Clinical cure rate	304 (2)	1.31 [0.74, 2.33]	Very low	Risk of bias, imprecision	There may be little or no difference in the clinical cure rate.
Development of resistant bacteria	0 (0)	-	-	-	No data available
Length of hospital stay	117 (1)	-	Very low	Risk of bias, imprecision, indirectness	There may be little or no difference in the length of stay.
Recurrence rate	187 (1)	-	Low	Imprecision, indirectness	There may be little or no difference in the rate of recurrence.
Adverse effect rate	176 (1)	-	Low	Imprecision, indirectness	There may be little or no difference in the rate of adverse effects.

CI: confidence interval, GRADE: GRADE Working Group grades of evidence.

4. Discussion

The current systematic review revealed a lack of evidence on anaerobic coverage for aspiration pneumonia; only one randomised trial and two observational studies were found eligible for the review. Although very limited in number, these publications did not show a clear benefit of anaerobic coverage in the treatment of patients diagnosed with aspiration pneumonia. No included studies reported benefit of anaerobic coverage in improving mortality.

When considering the need for anaerobic coverage, we must first understand the role of anaerobes in the development of aspiration pneumonia. Two factors, the overestimation and underestimation of their virulence, should be considered.

Previously, the high presence of anaerobes in lower respiratory tract specimens from patients with aspiration pneumonia led to the practice of covering anaerobes for their treatment [4–6]. The reported rate of identification of anaerobes in respiratory specimens from patients with aspiration pneumonia was as high as 73.9–100%. Treatment with agents covering anaerobes was often recommended [25,26].

However, since the 1990s, there has been a sharp downward trend in the detection of anaerobes in patients with aspiration pneumonia. The cause of this shift is suspected to be partly due to earlier sampling and intervention. Data reported in the 1970s showing a high prevalence of anaerobic organisms were often derived from samples taken late in the course of the disease [4–6,27]. Studies of more acute phase pneumonia have shown less impact of anaerobes [8,28–30]. Another consideration is the change in oral hygiene levels over the years. Oral health status is thought to have improved in recent decades, due in part to the advocacy of routine oral care [31]. There have been reports of improvements over the years in general oral status [32], number of missing teeth [33], and toothbrushing frequency [34]. The improvement in oral health is thought to have affected the oral microbiota and the causative organisms of aspiration pneumonia. Other suspected causes include changes in the demographic characteristics of patients [9], as study populations have shifted from relatively young patients with alcoholism or general anaesthesia to older patients. These changes may have contributed to the decrease in anaerobes being identified as pathogens.

Alternatively, despite advances in microbial testing methods, not all pathogens are identified. Anaerobes are known to be difficult to obtain and culture. Therefore, the fact that anaerobes are not identified does not rule out their possibility of being the causative organism. This risk of underestimating the involvement of anaerobes may lead to undertreatment, putting the patient at risk of prolonged illness, treatment failure, and death. Of the three studies included in this review, two used blood/sputum cultures and urine antigens to investigate the causative organism [20,23]. One study did not report any bacteriological analyses [21]. None of the studies reported a method to isolate anaerobes and the results do not mention the identification of anaerobes. Therefore, the risk of underestimating anaerobic involvement must be considered.

Furthermore, the identification of an organism from the respiratory tract does not automatically define it as the cause of active infection. The virulence of anaerobes is not always high [3,4]. Overestimation of microbiological results leads to unnecessary antimicrobial coverage, with the risk of adverse events and complications such as C. difficile infection, and a burden on healthcare costs. In addition, not all anaerobes require additional empirical anaerobic coverage with beta-lactams or clindamycin [30]. The shift in oral anaerobes also suggests that common anaerobes causing aspiration pneumonia may be susceptible to routine CAP treatment [19], although the clinical scenario must also be taken into account [15]. Therefore, even in cases where anaerobes are thought to be the cause of aspiration pneumonia, this does not automatically justify the use of specific antibiotics to cover them.

The definition of aspiration pneumonia is not well established. Although there is a common understanding that aspiration pneumonia is a pneumonia in people with risk factors or signs of aspiration [35], there are no robust criteria. The reported ratio of aspiration pneumonia in community-acquired pneumonia ranges from 5.6% to over 90% [1,36,37] and is highly variable depending on the setting, population, and local understanding of the disease.

Among the studies included in this review, Oi et al. included patients who were diagnosed with CAP/NHCAP who were at risk of aspiration [23], Hasegawa et al. included pneumonia with an aspiration-related risk factor [21], and Marumo et al. included aspiration pneumonia in the NHCAP group B (no risk of MDR pathogen) [20]. The diagnosis of aspiration pneumonia in the presence of one risk factor (such as a history of stroke) is one of the broader definitions [35], compared with others that assess more factors such as swallowing function or pneumonia distribution. If patients with CAP are overly being diagnosed as aspiration pneumonia, this may lead to an underestimation of the role of anaerobes and necessity of anaerobic coverage. While a broad diagnosis of aspiration pneumonia may be meaningful in clinical practice (in order to prevent overlooking the possibility of an aspiration and to assess risk factors and swallowing function carefully), the risk of overdiagnosis cannot be denied in the current context of research. For research purposes, it is necessary to have a common definition of aspiration pneumonia.

Not all risk factors for aspiration are uniformly associated with aspiration pneumonia; rather, the degree to which they cause the disease is thought to vary. For example, in a recent study, of the common risk factors for aspiration pneumonia, impaired consciousness was the most closely associated with chest images suggestive of aspiration pneumonia [38]. Labelling patients with CAP/NHCAP with any risk factor of aspiration as 'aspiration pneumonia' may result in the concept of the disease being too broad.

The current suggested approach is to consider aspiration pneumonia not as a distinct entity, but as a continuum of community or hospital acquired pneumonia [9,39,40]. As the associated risk factors and degree of aspiration vary within the spectrum of aspiration pneumonia, the need for anaerobic coverage is also expected to vary.

Current treatment recommendations by various guidelines are highly dependent on observational studies, and varies between regions [17]. The ATS/IDSA guidelines recommend that anaerobic coverage should not be routinely added for suspected aspiration pneumonia unless lung abscess or empyema is suspected [14]. This is mainly based on observational studies reporting a decrease in the detection of anaerobes as causative organisms [28–30]. Our systematic review and meta-analysis are in line with these publications, and add interventional evidence to this view.

Our review shows that, according to the current literature, anaerobic coverage may not always be beneficial in the treatment of aspiration pneumonia. Anaerobic coverage may be unnecessary for initial empiric treatment in the absence of abscess formation or empyema and with good oral hygiene. Further management should be based not merely on the diagnostic labelling, but through consideration of patient history, comorbidities, level of consciousness, oral health, previous and current microbiology results, local antibiogram data, previous treatment and nursing/medical care, severity, chest imaging results, and response to treatment [41,42].

There are some limitations in this study that should be mentioned. This review focused on aspiration pneumonia. As the definition varies between settings [35], studies that did not mention the term 'aspiration' may not have been identified in the search process. Therefore, we performed manual searches of guidelines and references of relevant papers to identify related articles that may have been missed in the database searches, and added 'necrotising pneumonia' and 'lung abscess' to our search terms. Despite adding these terms to the search strategy, none of the included studies mentioned whether their participants had necrotising pneumonia or lung abscess. Nevertheless, caution should be taken in interpreting the results, as aspiration pneumonia is still a variable term. Additionally, the included studies all originated from Japan. However, as there was no restriction on the year or country of publication, this is a reflection of the characteristics of the current literature. It is possible that there are differences compared with other countries, although local data do not support this [39]. In addition, the antimicrobials selected in the studies were not uniform. Therefore, no general recommendation can be made from this result. As this is an issue of high clinical importance, further research is needed on the optimal antibiotic treatment of aspiration pneumonia and how to select those who may benefit from anaerobic coverage.

5. Conclusions

In the current review, no clear evidence was found to recommend routine anaerobic coverage for the antibiotic treatment of aspiration pneumonia. There are insufficient data to assess the necessity of anaerobic coverage. Further studies are needed to determine which cases of aspiration pneumonia require anaerobic coverage, if any.

Author Contributions: Conceptualisation, Y.Y., K.K. and S.T.; methodology, Y.Y., M.A., K.K., S.H. and Y.N.; formal analysis, Y.Y., M.A. and K.K.; investigation, Y.Y., M.A., S.H. and Y.N.; resources, Y.Y. and M.A.; data curation, Y.Y. and M.A.; writing—original draft preparation, Y.Y.; writing—review and editing, K.K., M.M., F.H., K.S. and S.T.; visualisation, M.A., S.H. and Y.N.; supervision, K.K., M.M., F.H., K.S. and S.T.; project administration, Y.Y. and K.K. All authors have read and agreed to the published version of the manuscript.

Funding: This research received no external funding.

Institutional Review Board Statement: Not applicable.

Informed Consent Statement: Not applicable.

Data Availability Statement: All relevant data are within the manuscript.

Acknowledgments: The authors would like to express their sincere gratitude to Nobuyuki Horita and the committee members of The Japanese Respiratory Society guidelines in management of adult pneumonia on their guidance in this study.

Conflicts of Interest: Yuki Yoshimatsu is supported by The Japanese Respiratory Society Fellowship Grant. This review was supported by the Japanese Respiratory Society as part of the process of developing their newest pneumonia guidelines. The authors received no financial support for the research, authorship, and publication of this article. The authors declare that they have no other competing interests. The funders had no role in the design of the study; in the collection, analyses, or interpretation of data; in the writing of the manuscript; or in the decision to publish the results.

Appendix A

Appendix A.1. Search Strategy for PubMED

("pneumonia, aspiration"[mh] OR "respiratory aspiration"[mh] OR "aspiration pneumon*"[tw]) OR (pneumonia[mh] AND aspiration[tiab]) AND ("anti-bacterial agents"[tw] OR "anti-bacterial agents"[mh] OR antibiotic[tw] OR antimicrobial[tw] OR treatment[tiab]) NOT ("animals"[MeSH Terms] NOT "humans"[MeSH Terms]) AND (Randomized Controlled Trial[pt] OR Adaptive Clinical Trial[pt] OR Clinical Trial[pt] OR Clinical Trial, Phase*[pt] OR Comparative Study[pt] OR Controlled Clinical Trial[pt] OR Equivalence Trial[pt] OR Evaluation Study[pt] OR Multicenter Study[pt] OR Observational Study[pt] OR Validation Study[pt] OR Clinical Study[pt] OR Pragmatic Clinical Trial[pt] OR case control study[tw] OR Randomized Controlled Trial[tw] OR Adaptive Clinical Trial[tw] OR Clinical Trial[tw] OR Clinical Trial, Phase*[tw] OR Comparative Study[tw] OR Controlled Clinical Trial[tw] OR Equivalence Trial[tw] OR Evaluation Study[tw] OR Multicenter Study[tw] OR Observational Study[tw] OR Validation Study[tw] OR Clinical Study[tw] OR Pragmatic Clinical Trial[tw] or control*[tw] or cohort[tw] or prospective*[tw]).

Appendix A.2. Search Strategy for Cochrane

([mh "pneumonia, aspiration"] OR [mh "respiratory aspiration"] OR ("aspiration" NEXT pneumon*):ti,ab,kw) OR ([mh pneumonia] AND aspiration:ti,ab) AND ("anti-bacterial agents":ti,ab,kw OR [mh "anti-bacterial agents"] OR antibiotic:ti,ab,kw OR antimicrobial:ti,ab,kw OR treatment:ti,ab) NOT ([mh animals] NOT [mh humans]) AND ("Randomized Controlled Trial":pt OR "Adaptive Clinical Trial":pt OR "Clinical Trial":pt OR ("Clinical Trial," NEXT Phase*):pt OR "Comparative Study":pt OR "Controlled Clinical Trial":pt OR "Equivalence Trial":pt OR "Evaluation Study":pt OR "Multicenter Study":pt OR "Observational Study":pt OR "Validation Study":pt OR "Clinical Study":pt OR "Pragmatic Clinical Trial":pt OR "case control study":ti,ab,kw OR "Randomized Controlled Trial":ti,ab,kw OR "Adaptive Clinical Trial":ti,ab,kw OR "Clinical Trial":ti,ab,kw OR ("Clinical Trial," NEXT Phase*):ti,ab,kw OR "Comparative Study":ti,ab,kw OR "Controlled Clinical Trial":ti,ab,kw OR "Equivalence Trial":ti,ab,kw OR "Evaluation Study":ti,ab,kw

OR "Multicenter Study":ti,ab,kw OR "Observational Study":ti,ab,kw OR "Validation Study":ti,ab,kw OR "Clinical Study":ti,ab,kw OR "Pragmatic Clinical Trial":ti,ab,kw OR control*:ti,ab,kw OR cohort:ti,ab,kw OR prospective*:ti,ab,kw).

Appendix A.3. Funnel Plots for Publication Bias Evaluation

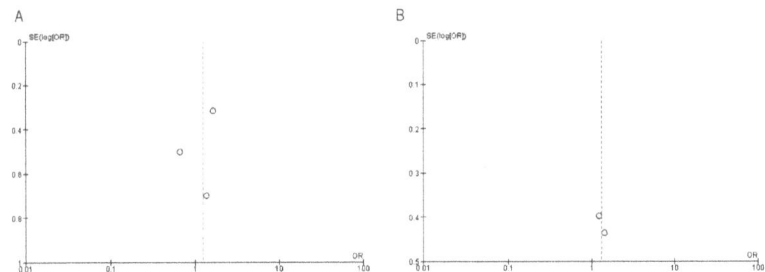

Figure A1. Funnel plots. (**A**) Mortality, (**B**) Clinical cure rate.

References

1. Teramoto, S.; Fukuchi, Y.; Sasaki, H.; Sato, K.; Sekizawa, K.; Matsuse, T. High incidence of aspiration pneumonia in community- and hospital-acquired pneumonia in hospitalized patients: A multicenter, prospective study in Japan. *J. Am. Geriatr. Soc.* **2008**, *56*, 577–579. [CrossRef] [PubMed]
2. Komiya, K.; Ishii, H.; Umeki, K.; Mizunoe, S.; Okada, F.; Johkoh, T.; Kadota, J. Impact of aspiration pneumonia in patients with com-munity-acquired pneumonia and healthcare-associated pneumonia: A multicenter retrospective cohort study. *Respirology* **2013**, *18*, 514–521. [CrossRef] [PubMed]
3. Bartlett, J.G. How Important Are Anaerobic Bacteria in Aspiration Pneumonia: When Should They Be Treated and What Is Optimal Therapy. *Infect. Dis. Clin. N. Am.* **2013**, *27*, 149–155. [CrossRef] [PubMed]
4. Bartlett, J.G.; Gorbach, S.L.; Finegold, S.M. The bacteriology of aspiration pneumonia. *Am. J. Med.* **1974**, *56*, 202–207. [CrossRef]
5. Cesar, L.; Gonzalez, C.; Calia, F.M. Bacteriologic flora of aspiration-induced pulmonary infections. *Arch Intern Med.* **1975**, *135*, 711–714. [CrossRef]
6. Lorber, B.; Swenson, R.M. Bacteriology of aspiration pneumonia. A prospective study of community- and hospital-acquired cases. *Ann. Intern. Med.* **1974**, *81*, 329–331. [CrossRef]
7. Finegold, S.M. Anaerobic bacteria. Their role in infection and their management. *Postgrad. Med.* **1987**, *81*, 141–147. [CrossRef]
8. Marin-Corral, J.; Pascual-Guardia, S.; Amati, F.; Aliberti, S.; Masclans, J.R.; Soni, N.; Rodriguez, A.; Sibila, O.; Sanz, F.; Sotgiu, G.; et al. Aspiration Risk Factors, Microbiology, and Empiric Antibiotics for Patients Hospitalized with Community-Acquired Pneumonia. *Chest* **2021**, *159*, 58–72. [CrossRef]
9. Mandell, L.A.; Niederman, M.S. Aspiration Pneumonia. *N. Engl. J. Med.* **2019**, *380*, 651–663. [CrossRef]
10. Metlay, J.P.; Waterer, G.W.; Long, A.C.; Anzueto, A.; Brozek, J.; Crothers, K.; Cooley, L.A.; Dean, N.C.; Fine, M.J.; Flanders, S.A.; et al. Diagnosis and treatment of adults with community-acquired pneumonia. An official clinical practice guideline of the american thoracic society and infectious diseases society of America. *Am. J. Respir. Crit. Care Med.* **2019**, *200*, e45–e67. [CrossRef]
11. Lim, W.S.; Baudouin, S.V.; George, R.C.; Hill, A.T.; Jamieson, C.; Le Jeune, I.; Macfarlane, J.T.; Read, R.C.; Roberts, H.J.; Levy, M.L.; et al. BTS guidelines for the management of community acquired pneumonia in adults: Update 2009. *Thorax* **2009**, *64*, iii1–iii55. [CrossRef] [PubMed]
12. Chanderraj, R.; Baker, J.M.; Kay, S.G.; Brown, C.A.; Hinkle, K.J.; Fergle, D.J.; McDonald, R.A.; Falkowski, N.R.; Metcalf, J.D.; Kaye, K.S.; et al. In critically ill patients, anti-anaerobic antibiotics increase risk of adverse clinical outcomes. *Eur. Respir. J.* **2023**, *61*, 2200910. [CrossRef] [PubMed]
13. Simeonova, M.; Daneman, N.; Lam, P.W.; Elligsen, M. Addition of anaerobic coverage for treatment of biliary tract infections: A propensity score-matched cohort study. *JAC Antimicrob. Resist.* **2023**, *5*, dlac141. [CrossRef] [PubMed]
14. Rodriguez, A.E.; Restrepo, M.I. New perspectives in aspiration community acquired Pneumonia. *Expert Rev. Clin. Pharmacol.* **2019**, *12*, 991–1002. [CrossRef] [PubMed]
15. DiBardino, D.M.; Wunderink, R.G. Aspiration pneumonia: A review of modern trends. *J. Crit. Care* **2015**, *30*, 40–48. [CrossRef]
16. Page, M.; McKenzie, J.; Bossuyt, P.; Boutron, I.; Hoffmann, T.; Mulrow, C.; Shamseer, L.; Tetzlaff, J.; Akl, E.; Brennan, S.; et al. The PRISMA 2020 statement: An updated guideline for reporting systematic reviews. *BMJ* **2021**, *372*, n71. [CrossRef]
17. The Japanese Respiratory Society. *The JRS Guidelines for the Management of Pneumonia in Adults*; Medical Review Co.: Tokyo, Japan, 2017.
18. Klompas, M. Aspiration Pneumonia in Adults. UpToDate. 2022. Available online: https://www.uptodate.com/contents/aspiration-pneumonia-in-adults (accessed on 15 September 2022).
19. Bowerman, T.J.; Zhang, J.; Waite, L.M. Antibacterial treatment of aspiration pneumonia in older people: A systematic review. *Clin. Interv. Aging* **2018**, *13*, 2201–2213. [CrossRef]

20. Marumo, S.; Teranishi, T.; Higami, Y.; Koshimo, Y.; Kiyokawa, H.; Kato, M. Effectiveness of azithromycin in aspiration pneumonia: A prospective observational study. *BMC Infect. Dis.* **2014**, *14*, 685. [CrossRef]
21. Hasegawa, S.; Shiraishi, A.; Yaegashi, M.; Hosokawa, N.; Morimoto, K.; Mori, T. Ceftriaxone versus ampicillin/sulbactam for the treatment of aspiration-associated pneumonia in adults. *J. Comp. Eff. Res.* **2019**, *8*, 1275–1284. [CrossRef]
22. Wells, G.A.; Shea, B.; O'Connell, D.; Peterson, J.; Welch, V.; Losos, M.; Tugwell, P. The Newcastle-Ottawa Scale (NOS) for Assessing the Quality of Nonrandomised Studies in Meta-Analyses. Available online: http://www.ohri.ca/programs/clinical_epidemiology/oxford.asp (accessed on 16 December 2019).
23. Oi, I.; Ito, I.; Tanabe, N.; Konishi, S.; Hamao, N.; Yasutomo, Y.; Kadowaki, S.; Hirai, T. Cefepime vs. meropenem for moderate-to-severe pneumonia in patients at risk for aspiration: An open-label, randomized study. *J. Infect. Chemother.* **2020**, *26*, 181–187. [CrossRef]
24. Sterne, J.A.C.; Savović, J.; Page, M.J.; Elbers, R.G.; Blencowe, N.S.; Boutron, I.; Cates, C.J.; Cheng, H.Y.; Corbett, M.S.; Eldridge, S.M.; et al. RoB 2: A revised tool for assessing risk of bias in randomised trials. *BMJ* **2019**, *366*, l4898. [CrossRef] [PubMed]
25. Bartlett, J.G.; Gorbach, S.L. Treatment of aspiration pneumonia and primary lung abscess. Penicillin G vs clindamycin. *JAMA* **1975**, *234*, 935–937. [CrossRef] [PubMed]
26. Lode, H. Microbiological and clinical aspects of aspiration pneumonia. *J. Antimicrob. Chemother.* **1988**, *21*, 83–90. [CrossRef] [PubMed]
27. Marik, P.E. Aspiration Pneumonitis and Aspiration Pneumonia. *N. Engl. J. Med.* **2001**, *344*, 665–671. [CrossRef] [PubMed]
28. El-Solh, A.A.; Pietrantoni, C.; Bhat, A.; Aquilina, A.T.; Okada, M.; Grover, V.; Gifford, N. Microbiology of Severe Aspiration Pneumonia in Institutionalized Elderly. *Am. J. Respir. Crit. Care Med.* **2003**, *167*, 1650–1654. [CrossRef]
29. Marik, P.E.; Careau, P. The role of anaerobes in patients with ventilator-associated pneumonia and aspiration pneumonia: A prospective study. *Chest* **1999**, *115*, 178–183. [CrossRef] [PubMed]
30. Mier, L.; Dreyfuss, D.; Darchy, B.; Lanore, J.J.; Djedaini, K.; Weber, P.; Brun, P.; Coste, F. Is penicillin G an adequate initial treatment for aspiration pneumonia? A prospective evaluation using a protected specimen brush and quantitative cultures. *Intensive Care Med.* **1993**, *19*, 279–284. [CrossRef]
31. Yoneyama, T.; Yoshida, M.; Matsui, T.; Sasaki, H. Oral care and pneumonia. Oral Care Working Group. *Lancet* **1999**, *354*, 515. [CrossRef]
32. Kocher, T.; Holtfreter, B.; Pitchika, V.; Kuhr, K.; Jordan, R.A. Trends in dental and oral health status in Germany between 1997 and 2014. *Bundesgesundheitsblatt Gesundh. Gesundheitsschutz* **2021**, *64*, 782–792. [CrossRef]
33. Furuta, M.; Takeuchi, K.; Takeshita, T.; Shibata, Y.; Suma, S.; Kageyama, S.; Asakawa, M.; Hata, J.; Yoshida, D.; Shimazaki, Y.; et al. 10-year trend of tooth loss and associated factors in a Japanese population-based longitudinal study. *BMJ Open* **2021**, *11*, e048114. [CrossRef]
34. Raittio, E.; Helakorpi, S.; Suominen, A.L. Age-Period-Cohort Analysis of Toothbrushing Frequency in Finnish Adults: Results from Annual National Cross-Sectional Surveys From 1978 to 2014. *Int. Dent. J.* **2021**, *71*, 233–241. [CrossRef] [PubMed]
35. Yoshimatsu, Y.; Melgaard, D.; Westergren, A.; Skrubbeltrang, C.; Smithard, D.G. The diagnosis of aspiration pneumonia in older persons: A systematic review. *Eur. Geriatr. Med.* **2022**, *13*, 1071–1080. [CrossRef] [PubMed]
36. Marrie, T.J.; Durant, H.; Yates, L. Community-Acquired Pneumonia Requiring Hospitalization: 5-Year Prospective Study. *Rev. Infect. Dis.* **1989**, *11*, 586–599. [CrossRef] [PubMed]
37. Komiya, K.; Ishii, H.; Kadota, J.-I. Healthcare-associated Pneumonia and Aspiration Pneumonia. *Aging Dis.* **2015**, *6*, 27–37. [CrossRef] [PubMed]
38. Komiya, K.; Yamamoto, T.; Yoshikawa, H.; Goto, A.; Umeki, K.; Johkoh, T.; Hiramatsu, K.; Kadota, J.-I. Factors associated with gravity-dependent dis-tribution on chest CT in elderly patients with community-acquired pneumonia: A retrospective observational study. *Sci. Rep.* **2022**, *12*, 8023. [CrossRef] [PubMed]
39. Yoshimatsu, Y.; Smithard, D.G. A Paradigm Shift in the Diagnosis of Aspiration Pneumonia in Older Adults. *J. Clin. Med.* **2022**, *11*, 5214. [CrossRef]
40. Smithard, D.G.; Yoshimatsu, Y. Pneumonia, Aspiration Pneumonia, or Frailty-Associated Pneumonia? *Geriatrics* **2022**, *7*, 115. [CrossRef]
41. Yoshimatsu, Y.; Tobino, K.; Ko, Y.; Yasuda, M.; Ide, H.; Oku, Y. Careful history taking detects initially unknown underlying causes of aspiration pneumonia. *Geriatr. Gerontol. Int.* **2020**, *20*, 785–790. [CrossRef]
42. Yoshimatsu, Y.; Tobino, K.; Ortega, O.; Oda, H.; Ota, H.; Kawabata, T.; Hiramatsu, K.; Murakami, Y.; Clavé, P. Development and implementation of an aspiration pneumonia cause investigation algorithm. *Clin. Respir. J.* **2022**, *17*, 20–28. [CrossRef]

Disclaimer/Publisher's Note: The statements, opinions and data contained in all publications are solely those of the individual author(s) and contributor(s) and not of MDPI and/or the editor(s). MDPI and/or the editor(s) disclaim responsibility for any injury to people or property resulting from any ideas, methods, instructions or products referred to in the content.

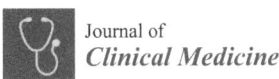

Article

Use of Maximum Tongue Pressure Values to Examine the Presence of Dysphagia after Extubation and Prevent Aspiration Pneumonia in Elderly Emergency Patients

Ryo Ichibayashi [1], Hideki Sekiya [2,*], Kosuke Kaneko [2] and Mitsuru Honda [1]

[1] Department of Critical Care Center, Toho University Medical Center Omori Hospital, Tokyo 143-8541, Japan
[2] Department of Oral Surgery, School of Medicine, Toho University, Tokyo 143-8541, Japan
* Correspondence: sekiya-h@med.toho-u.ac.jp

Abstract: Background: Tongue pressure values in patients with dysphagia are reported to be significantly lower than those in healthy controls. The aim of this study was to measure the maximum tongue pressure (MTP) values after extubation in order to assess the presence of post-extubation dysphagia for the safe initiation of oral intake in elderly patients. Methods: Data from 90 patients who were extubated after mechanical ventilation under tracheal intubation were collected retrospectively. The patients were divided into two groups as follows: normal group (those who did not develop aspiration pneumonia after extubation; median age 62 years) and aspiration group (those who developed aspiration during the evaluation period; median age 75 years). The MTP values were measured at 6 h, 24 h, 3 days, and 7 days after extubation. Results: The values were significantly increased 24 h after extubation in the normal group ($p < 0.05$). Alternatively, no increase was observed even after 1 week of extubation in the aspiration group, and the values were significantly lower than those in the normal group. The cutoff values at 6 and 24 h after extubation, which were measured using the receiver operator characteristic (ROC) curve, were 17.8 and 23.2 kpa, respectively; furthermore, the results of these assessments were strongly related to the development of aspiration 6 h after extubation (χ^2-value: 6.125; $p = 0.0133$). Conclusions: The presence of post-extubation dysphagia in patients who are intubated for ≥24 h can be predicted based on age and the MTP values at 6 h after extubation.

Keywords: post-extubation; aspiration pneumonia; dysphagia; maximum tongue pressure (MTP); oral intake; rehabilitation; elderly emergency patients

Citation: Ichibayashi, R.; Sekiya, H.; Kaneko, K.; Honda, M. Use of Maximum Tongue Pressure Values to Examine the Presence of Dysphagia after Extubation and Prevent Aspiration Pneumonia in Elderly Emergency Patients. *J. Clin. Med.* 2022, 11, 6599. https://doi.org/10.3390/jcm11216599

Academic Editor: César Picado

Received: 1 October 2022
Accepted: 3 November 2022
Published: 7 November 2022

Publisher's Note: MDPI stays neutral with regard to jurisdictional claims in published maps and institutional affiliations.

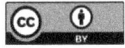

Copyright: © 2022 by the authors. Licensee MDPI, Basel, Switzerland. This article is an open access article distributed under the terms and conditions of the Creative Commons Attribution (CC BY) license (https://creativecommons.org/licenses/by/4.0/).

1. Introduction

Approximately half of all patients receiving mechanical ventilation with endotracheal intubation experience post-extubation dysphagia [1–3]. Older adults and those with underlying diseases might experience pre-existing dysphagia; therefore, the assessment of swallowing function in individuals who have been transported to the emergency department is challenging. Although researchers have speculated that muscle weakness and sensory impairment due to long-term intubation can cause dysphagia after tracheal intubation, no definitive conclusions have been reached so far [4]. Prolonged hospitalization and poor prognosis are common in patients who experience dysphagia after extubation, and could lead to increased medical expenses [5].

Several screening methods, such as the repetitive saliva swallowing test, modified water swallowing test, and other bedside evaluations, can be used to assess tongue movement and the oral environment in order to determine the presence of dysphagia [6]. However, despite the use of these methods, dysphagia can remain undiagnosed in some patients and lead to aspiration or pneumonia. The tongue pressure test is a quantitative measure of the swallowing ability, wherein a numerical value is assigned to assess the tongue function [7–9]. Previous studies have indicated that tongue pressure is associated with dysphagia; tongue pressure values in patients with dysphagia were reported to be significantly lower in patients with dysphagia than those in healthy controls, and were correlated with other well-known functional criteria used to evaluate the swallowing ability [9,10]. A maximum value of <30 kPa indicates decreased tongue pressure and might reveal the presence of dysphagia [11]. Tongue pressure measurements are easy to obtain owing to the noninvasive nature of the method used during bedside evaluations of the swallowing function after extubation; additionally, this method yields reproducible quantitative values [12]. The aim of the present study was to measure the maximum tongue pressure (MTP) values in patients who underwent extubation in order to determine whether these values can be used to assess the presence of post-extubation dysphagia for the safe initiation of oral intake of foods.

2. Participants and Methods
2.1. Participants

The sample size required for this study was calculated assuming a 1:2 ratio of patients with and without post-extubation aspiration findings [5]. Therefore, data from a total of 93 patients were required to obtain an area under the curve (AUC) value calculated from the receiver operating characteristic (ROC) curve of ≥ 0.7 (power of detection 95%). Subsequently, data from 90 patients who were brought to the Emergency Life Support Center at our hospital from 2012 to 2016 were collected. Those who received mechanical ventilation with endotracheal intubation for 24 h or longer, and whose primary condition was successfully treated resulting in extubation, were included in the study. The exclusion criteria were as follows: cases where it was not possible to obtain regular measurements, patients who underwent re-intubation or experienced delirium within 7 days after extubation, and patients with neurologic/cerebrovascular disorders. All participants were evaluated by using the repetitive saliva swallowing test [13] and modified water swallowing test [6], and participants without dysphagia were initiated on oral intake. The participants without dysphagia resumed oral intake with the same form of food as before their ICU admission and swallowing rehabilitation from post-extubation to the start of oral intake consisted of indirect training as the usual protocol used in our hospital.

The present study was approved by the Toho University Medical Center Omori Hospital Ethics Committee. Written explanations regarding the aims and procedures used in the study were provided, and informed consent was obtained from all the participants or their family members prior to enrollment (Approval No. 24-132).

2.2. Methods and Data Collection

A TPM-01 device (JMS, Hiroshima, Japan) was used to measure the tongue pressure (Figure 1). The MTP values were measured at 6 h, 24 h, 3 days, and 7 days after extubation. The maximum values of three individual measurements collected at each time point were recorded in kPa. The actual measurements were obtained by a designated nurse at the Emergency and Critical Care Center, or by members of a specially trained swallowing support team in the regular wards. All evaluators received specific instructions regarding the tongue pressure measurements to ensure inter-observer reliability.

The characteristics of the patients, including age, sex, tracheal intubation period, Acute Physiology and Chronic Health Evaluation II (APACHE II) score, and causative disease, were retrospectively evaluated. The patients were divided into two groups as follows: those who did not develop aspiration pneumonia after extubation (normal group) and those who developed aspiration during the evaluation period, resulting in aspiration pneumonia or signs of aspiration pneumonia with the cessation of oral intake (aspiration group). Newly or recurrent visible infiltrative shadows on recent radiographs obtained from the medical records were required for signs of aspiration pneumonia. In addition, the ability to use the MTP values obtained at 6 and 24 h after extubation to assess dysphagia in order to predict the optimum time for the safe initiation of oral intake in the normal and aspiration groups was examined. These values were chosen owing to the retrospective nature of this study, in order to adjust for the background characteristics before starting the oral intake. Oral intake was initiated 24 h after extubation at the discretion of the attending physician, but the MTP values were not used to determine whether the patients were ready to start the oral intake at that time.

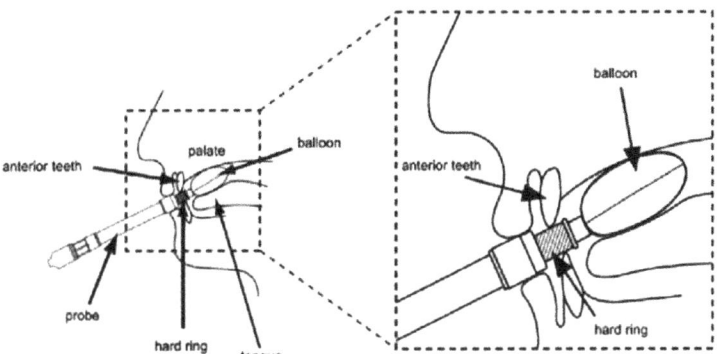

Figure 1. The method used to measure the tongue pressure [14]. The internal pressure of the balloon was adjusted to a predetermined pressure, after which it was positioned in the oral cavity as shown. The tongue pressure was measured by asking the patient to lift the tongue toward the palate with as much force as possible, as if to crush the balloon.

Since the primary endpoint of this study is the prediction of pneumonia at 24 h after extubation and after initiation of oral intake, data on MTP value at days 3 and 7 are presented as a secondary endpoint to the results.

2.3. Statistical Analysis

EZR ver1.52 (Kanda, 2014, Saitama, Japan [15]) was used for statistical analysis. The Mann–Whitney U-test was used to analyze differences in age, intubation time, and APACHE II scores, whereas the Chi-square test was used to examine differences in the male-female ratio and the causative diseases. Associations with MTP values after extubation were analyzed using the Friedman's test or Dunn's multiple comparison test. The MTP values at 6 h, 24 h, 3 days, and 7 days after extubation were compared between the normal and aspiration groups using the Mann–Whitney U-test. In addition, ROC curve analysis was performed to examine the MTP values at 6 and 24 h after extubation, in order to determine whether these values can be used to predict aspiration. The AUC values and the diagnostic cutoff value for MTP at 6 and 24 h were calculated from the ROC curves using Youden's J statistic. Statistical analyses of the ROC curve were performed also using EZR ver1.52.

Subsequently, a multivariable logistic regression analysis was performed to calculate the result. The objective variable for the analysis was the detection of aspiration pneumonia, and the explanatory variables were "Age above 75", "Causative diseases", "Low MTP value (6 h)", and "Low MTP value (24 h)". Data pertaining to age were categorized into groups (those younger than 75 years and above 75), because the age of the normal group was 75.6 years which is 1 SD more than the mean age. The median age of the aspiration group was 75 years, and this is due to the fact that the elderly classification in Japan is 75 years old or older. Causative diseases of intubation were classified into two groups. One group consisted of pneumonia, sepsis, exacerbation of chronic obstructive pulmonary disease (COPD), and acute pancreatitis, which cause ARDS; the other group consisted of other diseases. The MTP values at 6 and 24 h were classified as "low" and "high", respectively, as determined by their cutoff values. In addition, an ROC curve analysis was performed on the combined "Age above 63", "Low MTP value (6 h)", and "Low MTP value (24 h)".

A two-tailed p-value of <0.05 was considered statistically significant. The multivariable logistic regression analysis was also performed using EZR ver1.52.

The independent models were adjusted by confounders for the different times of the MTP using pair-matching analysis. We assumed age and causative disease as confounding factors. After correcting the confounding factors, the Mantel–Haenszel Chi-squared test with continuity correction was performed to examine the possibility of predicting aspiration at each time-point using EZR ver1.52.

3. Results

The normal and aspiration groups comprised 70 and 20 patients (22.2%), respectively; the background characteristics of the patients in the two groups are shown in Table 1. No significant differences in sex, endotracheal intubation period, or severity were observed between the groups. However, patients in the aspiration group were significantly older than those in the normal group ($p < 0.05$). Furthermore, no significant differences in the causative diseases for intubation were observed between the two groups (Table 2).

Table 1. Background characteristics of the patients in the normal and aspiration groups.

	Total ($n = 90$)	Normal ($n = 70$)	Aspiration ($n = 20$)	p-Value
Age (years); Average ± SD Median	62.9 ± 15.8 66	59.7 ± 15.9 62	73.9 ± 9.5 75	<0.01
Sex (male/female)	55/35	42/28	13/7	0.69
Intubation period (days) Average ± SD Median	8.1 ± 5.5 7	8.0 ± 5.8 6.5	8.5 ± 4.2 9	0.5
MTP value (at 6 h) Average ± SD Median	23.0 ± 10.1 21.6	24.8 ± 11.6 25.5	13.2 ± 7.5 13.9	<0.01
MTP value (at 24 h) Average ± SD Median	25.3 ± 11.7 24.9	24.9 ± 9.7 24.2	16.4 ± 8.8 18.7	<0.01
APACHE II score Average ± SD Median	23.9 ± 9.8 23	23.6 ± 10.0 22.5	24.8 ± 9.3 23	0.81

SD, standard deviation; APACHE II, Acute Physiology and Chronic Health Evaluation II.

Table 2. The disease background of the patients in the two groups.

	Normal ($n = 70$)	Aspiration ($n = 20$)	p-Value
CPA recovery	10	2	0.47
Trauma	5	1	0.60
Acute myocardial infarction	7	3	0.39
Heart failure	4	2	0.40
Pneumonia	13	6	0.21
Sepsis	7	4	0.20
Acute pancreatitis	2	0	0.44
COPD exacerbation	1	0	0.59
Others	21	2	0.07

CPA, cardiopulmonary arrest.

Changes in MTP values after extubation in the entire study population and in the two groups are shown in Figure 2. The MTP values were significantly ($p < 0.05$) increased to 20.7 kPa, 21.6 kPa, 24.9 kPa, and 26.7 kPa at 6 h, 24 h, 3 days, and 7 days after extubation, respectively, over a period of 1 week in the entire study population (Figure 2A). Similar findings were observed in the normal group (25.5 kPa, 24.2 kPa, 28.1 kPa, and 30.3 kPa at 6 h, 24 h, 3 days, and 7 days after extubation, respectively; Figure 2B). On the contrary, no significant increase was observed in the aspiration group, which exhibited significantly lower MTP values than those in the normal group (13.9 kPa, 18.7 kPa, 11.1 kPa, and 13.1 kPa at 6 h, 24 h, 3 days, and 7 days after extubation, respectively; Figure 2C). Significant differences in MTP values were observed between the groups at each time point (Figure 3). Multiple comparison tests revealed significant differences between the MTP values at 6 h and 3 days, 6 h and 7 days, 24 h and 3 days, and 24 h and 7 days ($p < 0.05$). No significant differences were observed between the 6- and 24-h mark ($p = 0.83$).

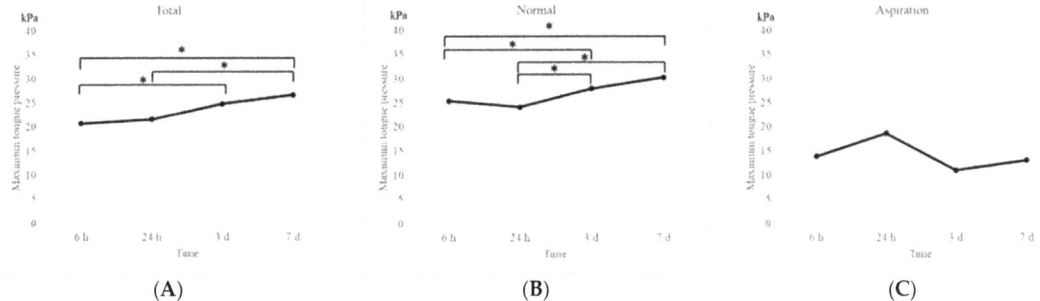

Figure 2. Graphs showing changes in MTP in the entire study population (**A**) and in the two groups (**B**,**C**). MTP values recovered over a period of 1 week after extubation in the entire study population (**A**) and the participants in the normal group ((**B**); Friedman test, $p < 0.05$). (**C**) The MTP values remained low even after 1 week in the aspiration group. * $p < 0.05$; h: hours; d: days. Friedman's test, Dunn's test.

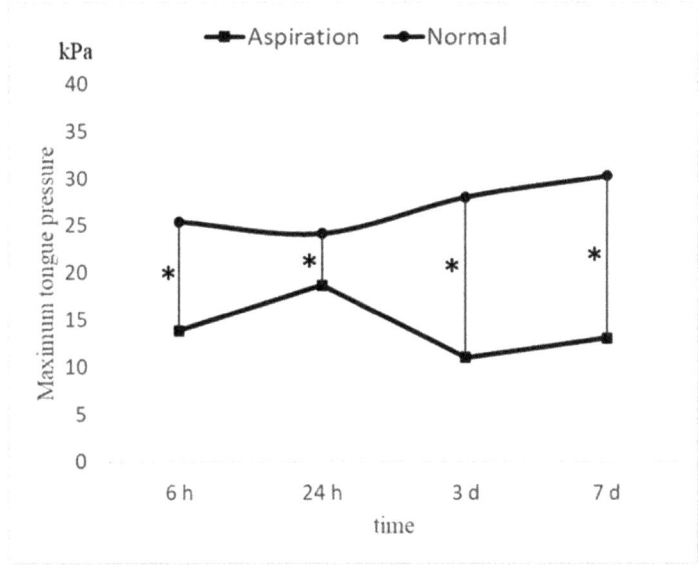

Figure 3. MTP values in the normal and aspiration groups. * $p < 0.05$; h: hours; d: days. Mann–Whitney U-test.

ROC curve analysis was performed to determine whether the MTP values after 6 and 24 h could be used to predict dysphagia. The diagnostic cutoff MTP value after 6 h was 17.8 kPa, the sensitivity was 80.0%, the specificity was 67.1%, the positive predictive value was 41.0%, and the negative predictive value was 92.2% (Figure 4A). The corresponding values (diagnostic cutoff, sensitivity, specificity, positive predictive, and negative predictive) after 24 h were 23.2 kPa, 90.0%, 52.9%, 35.3%, and 94.9%, respectively (Figure 4B).

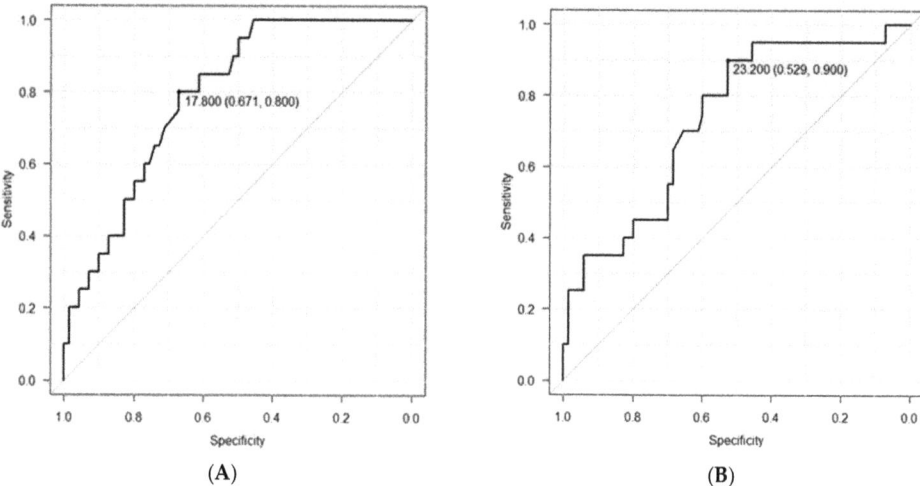

Figure 4. Receiver operating characteristic (ROC) curve analysis 6 and 24 h after extubation. (**A**) ROC curve analysis 6 h after extubation. (**B**) ROC curve analysis 24 h after extubation. It is possible to estimate diagnostic cutoff values from ROC curves.

The AUC values were calculated from the ROC curves using Youden's J statistic. The values after 6 h and 24 h were 0.79 (95% CI: 0.69–0.89) and 0.74 (95% CI: 0.61–0.86), respectively.

Multivariable logistic regression analysis was performed to determine the factors associated with aspiration after extubation (Table 3). "Age above 75" and "Low MTP value (6 h)" were the significant variables; therefore, ROC curve analysis was performed to investigate the predictive ability of the combination of "Age above 75", "Causative diseases", "Low MTP value (6 h)", and "Low MTP value (24 h)" for dysphagia (Figure 5). The AUC value was 0.81 (95% CI: 0.73–0.90).

We hypothesized that the combination of these items would aid in predicting post-extubation dysphagia, and "Age above 75" and "Causative diseases" were considered confounding factors. Therefore, a model excluding the confounding factors was created using the pair-matching analysis. A total of 40 cases, 20 in each of the two groups, was selected for the analysis (Table 4). The Mantel–Haenszel Chi-squared test was performed to examine the possibility of predicting aspiration at the 6 and 24 h time points, as shown in Table 5.

Table 3. Factors associated with aspiration after extubation by logistic regression analysis.

	Odds Ratio (95% CI)	*p*-Value
Age above 75	3.24 (1.01–10.4)	**0.048**
Causative diseases	0.472 (0.14–1.54)	0.214
Low MTP value (6 h)	4.25 (1.02–17.7)	**0.047**
Low MTP value (24 h)	3.26 (0.55–19.3)	0.194

CI: confidence interval. Bold: *p*-values indicate significance.

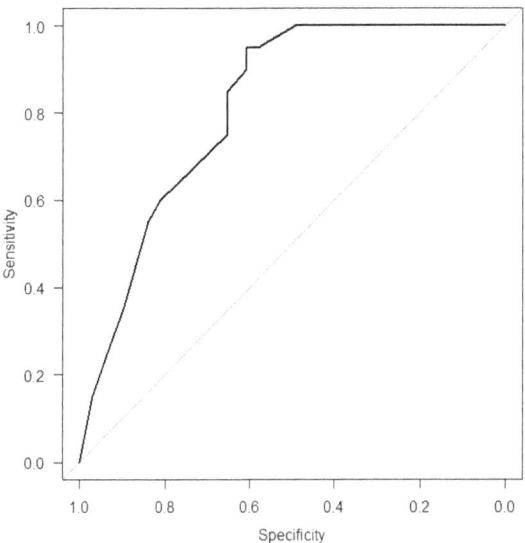

Figure 5. ROC curve analysis on the combined variables "Age above 75", "Causative diseases", "Low MTP value (6 h)", and "Low MTP value (24 h)". The AUC value was 0.81 (95% CI: 0.73–0.90).

Table 4. A new population excluding the confounding factors was created using the pair-matching analysis. A total of 40 cases, 20 in each in of the two groups, was selected for the analysis.

Age	Normal	Aspiration
<75 years	9	9
≥75 years	11	11
Causative Diseases	**Normal**	**Aspiration**
Pneumonia + ARDS Causal Diseases	9	9
Other	11	11

Table 5. The Mantel–Haenszel Chi-squared test with continuity correction was performed on each time point after correcting the confounding factors.

	χ^2-Value	p-Value
MTP value (at 6 h)	6.125	**0.0133**
MTP value (at 24 h)	2.50	0.1138

Bold: p-values indicate significance.

4. Discussion

The background factors were related to age in patients belonging to the normal and aspiration groups in this study; those in the aspiration group tended to be older than those in the normal group. The initiation of oral intake in elderly patients after life support should be approached with caution. Therefore, it is important to design an evaluation method that can be used to determine the optimum time for oral intake after extubation. No clear relationship was noted for either pneumonia or ARDS causal disease as the causative disease for intubation, which was speculated to be possibly related to post-extubation pneumonia. Prolonged endotracheal intubation is a common iatrogenic cause of swallowing disorders, but as shown in Table 1, there was no additional difference between the two groups ($p = 0.50$), so it was not included as a variable in the multivariate analysis.

This study included patients with severe disease (APACHE II: around 24), which is the reason for the higher incidence of pneumonia compared to previous reports [1–3].

The aim of the present study was to measure the MTP values in patients who underwent extubation in order to determine whether they can be used to assess the presence of post-extubation dysphagia, which could affect the initiation of oral intake in older patients. The participants in this study had normal RSST and modified water swallowing test results, so the development of post-extubation pneumonia or aspiration would be unlikely if true, but in 20 of the 90 cases, this occurred. This study suggests that post-extubation pneumonia due to dysphagia, which cannot be detected by conventional screening methods, may be predicted by using maximal tongue pressure in combination with conventional methods. Our findings indicated that the MTP values were initially low in patients requiring mechanical ventilation with endotracheal intubation for more than 24 h, but returned to normal levels after 1 week among those without dysphagia. These findings are in accordance with those of our previous study, which showed that patients with dysphagia exhibited lower MTP values, which did not significantly increase even after 1 week [14]. Evidence suggests that contact with the endotracheal tube during long-term oral intubation causes muscle weakness in the tongue and sensory impairment, leading to dysphagia; however, the underlying mechanisms remain unclear [4]. Early extubation and the use of appropriately-sized endotracheal tubes have been reported to reduce the risk of dysphagia [16]. However, other studies have reported no associations between the endotracheal intubation period and dysphagia [17].

Although no significant differences in MTP values were observed at 6 and 24 h after extubation in the normal group, the values were significantly increased after 3 days. It remains unclear as to why the MTP values did not recover within the first 24 h. Strict respiratory monitoring is required for at least 24–48 h after extubation [18] because hoarseness, laryngeal edema, and an increase in intraoral and sputum discharge caused by extubation can increase the risk of re-intubation during this period. Furthermore, the breathing effort is reported to increase, leading to fatigue of the respiratory muscles 1 h after extubation [19]. Heavy secretion in the oral cavity and increased sputum discharge are thought to delay the recovery of the swallowing function. Weakness of the swallowing muscles due to respiratory fatigue is known to continue for more than 24 h [20], which might account for the absence of any increase in the MTP value within the first 24 h after extubation. These findings highlight the importance of the respiratory status in relation to the swallowing function.

In the aspiration group, the MTP values did not recover 1 week after extubation; the MTP values were significantly lower in the aspiration group (13.9 kPa) than in the normal group (25.5 kPa) 6 h after extubation. Although the values had recovered to 18.7 kPa in the aspiration group 24 h after extubation in this study, they were below the normal values (30 kPa) [8,11]. Thus, it is important to measure the MTP value within 24 h of extubation to predict dysphagia.

The negative predictive values observed in the present study indicated that the ROC curve for MTP values could be used as an index for predicting aspiration 6 and 24 h after extubation. The diagnostic cutoff value of the MTP value after 6 h was 17.8 kPa, and the negative predictive value was 92.2%. The diagnostic cutoff value of the MTP value after 24 h was 23.2 kPa, and the negative predictive value was 94.9%. However, even if the MTP value is low, dysphagia may not necessarily be present. Thus, it may be necessary to evaluate other factors when examining the swallowing function following extubation. MTP values differ based on age and sex [8]. The findings of the current study suggest that age is a risk factor for aspiration after extubation. Tsai et al., reported that patients over 65 years of age are more likely to develop dysphagia after extubation, and should be monitored and treated for 1–2 weeks before resuming oral intake of food [21]. Older adults may exhibit a weak cough reflex or latent aspiration prior to hospitalization, which could increase the incidence of dysphagia due to tracheal intubation. Furthermore, various factors such as cognitive decline, a high incidence of delirium, and a history of taking multiple medications can increase the risk of aspiration in older adults.

Both age and pre-admission information regarding swallowing function are necessary to determine when oral intake can be re-initiated. Although it is difficult to obtain accurate information from the patient in the emergency department, our findings showed that MTP values 6 and 24 h after extubation were strongly associated with aspiration. Thus, when combined with other assessments, these values can be used to determine when oral intake can be initiated safely.

The average time for the re-initiation of oral intake after heart disease surgery is 118.4 h in patients with swallowing disorders [1]. The swallowing reflex can be restored within 1 week in patients who undergo long-term intubation in the intensive care unit (ICU) [22]. The length of hospitalization is extended in patients who develop swallowing disorders after extubation, thereby increasing the cost of treatment. The MTP values increased within 1 week after extubation in the present study; therefore, clinicians can use these values to determine the efficacy of rehabilitation and the time at which oral intake can be resumed after dysphagia, which could aid in shortening the hospitalization period and decreasing the treatment costs.

The results of this study indicate that 24 h after extubation, one can determine whether oral intake can be resumed. Oral intake can be safely initiated under the following conditions: in patients <75 years of age, when the MTP value is >17.8 kPa at 6 h after extubation, and the MTP value does not decrease after 24 h (remains > 23.2 kPa). In older emergency patients who do not meet these conditions, additional swallowing screening tests, videoendoscopy (VE) or videofluorography (VF), should be performed to diagnose the presence of dysphagia. Furthermore, the findings of this study suggest that regular measurement of the MTP is useful to determine the effectiveness of the rehabilitation and the appropriate time for resumption of oral intake.

In future studies, we need to design an interventional study in which patients with anticipated dysphagia determined by a new protocol with tongue pressure, were given rehabilitation prior to oral intake. We will then examine if the incidence of post-extubation pneumonia would decrease from 22%.

The MTP values may be of adjunctive use for other lung diseases, such as interstitial pneumonia with repeated acute conversions and dysphagia due to sarcopenia after COVID-19 infection [23]. Clinicians may find it challenging to determine the optimum time for the resumption of oral intake in patients with these diseases; thus, the use an ancillary tool other than the conventional swallowing assessment tests might prove beneficial.

5. Conclusions

This study demonstrated that the presence of post-extubation dysphagia can be assessed based on the MTP values at 6 and 24 h after extubation. This information can be used to determine the time for the initiation of oral intake in older emergency patients who have been intubated for ≥24 h. Additionally, changes in MTP values may be used to determine the optimum time when oral intake can be resumed and the efficacy of the rehabilitation following dysphagia. However, MTP values should be used in combination with other swallowing assessments to determine the most appropriate time for re-initiating oral intake. Additional study will be required to determine the most appropriate swallowing assessment that can be used in conjunction with MTP in the future.

Author Contributions: All authors were equally involved in the design, development, and conduct of the rapid review. R.I. wrote the first original draft of the manuscript and conducted the search, performed the statistics, preparation and submission of ethical documents and identified the list of articles. H.S. conducted the investigation, performed additional statistics and revised the manuscript based on feedback from all authors. K.K. was involved in data extraction. M.H. provided oversight and supervision. All authors have read and agreed to the published version of the manuscript.

Funding: This study was supported by the Japan Society for the Promotion of Science, Grant-in-Aid for Scientific Research (C) (Grant number: 22K10477) to H.S.

Institutional Review Board Statement: This study was conducted in accordance with the ethical guidelines for medical and health research involving human subjects and those for epidemiological research of the Ministry of Health, Labor and Welfare of Japan; approval for the study was obtained from the ethics committee of the Toho University Oomori Medical Center (Approval No. 24-132).

Informed Consent Statement: Informed consent was obtained from all participants or their family members after providing written explanations of the study goals and procedures and prior to enrollment in the study. The participants were informed of the right to refuse to participate in the study.

Data Availability Statement: The data presented in this study are available on request from the corresponding author. The data are not publicly available due to privacy and ethical considerations.

Acknowledgments: We would like to express our gratitude to the doctors in our department.

Conflicts of Interest: The authors declare that there is no conflict of interest in this study.

References

1. Barker, J.; Martino, R.; Reichardt, B.; Hickey, E.J.; Ralph-Edwards, A. Incidence and impact of dysphagia in patients receiving prolonged endotracheal intubation after cardiac surgery. *Can. J. Surg.* **2009**, *52*, 119–124. [PubMed]
2. Tolep, K.; Getch, C.L.; Criner, G.J. Swallowing dysfunction in patients receiving prolonged mechanical ventilation. *Chest* **1996**, *109*, 167–172. [CrossRef] [PubMed]
3. Ajemian, M.S.; Nirmul, G.B.; Anderson, M.T.; Zirlen, D.M.; Kwasnik, E.M. Routine fiberoptic endoscopic evaluation of swallowing following prolonged intubation. *Arch. Surg.* **2001**, *136*, 434–437. [CrossRef]
4. Su, H.; Hsiao, T.Y.; Ku, S.C.; Wang, T.G.; Lee, J.J.; Tzeng, W.C.; Huang, G.H.; Chen, C.C. Tongue weakness and somatosensory disturbance following oral endotracheal extubation. *Dysphagia* **2015**, *30*, 188–195. [CrossRef] [PubMed]
5. Macht, M.; Wimbish, T.; Bodine, C.; Moss, M. ICU-acquired swallowing disorders. *Crit. Care Med.* **2013**, *41*, 2396–2405. [CrossRef] [PubMed]
6. Tohara, H.; Saitoh, E.; Mays, K.A.; Kuhlemeier, K.; Palmer, J.B. Three tests for predicting aspiration without videofluorography. *Dysphagia* **2003**, *18*, 126–134. [CrossRef] [PubMed]
7. Hayashi, R.; Tsuga, K.; Hosokawa, R.; Yoshida, M.; Akagawa, Y. Novel handy probe for tongue pressure measurement. *Int. J. Prosthodont.* **2002**, *15*, 385–388. [PubMed]
8. Utanohara, Y.; Hayashi, R.; Yoshikawa, M.; Yoshida, M.; Akagawa, Y. Standard values of maximum tongue pressure taken using newly developed disposable tongue pressure measurement device. *Dysphagia* **2008**, *23*, 286–290. [CrossRef] [PubMed]
9. Tsuga, K.; Yoshikawa, M.; Oue, H.; Okazaki, Y.; Tsuchioka, H.; Maruyama, M.; Yoshida, M.; Akagawa, Y. Maximal voluntary tongue pressure is decreased in Japanese frail elderly persons. *Gerodontology* **2012**, *29*, 1078–1085. [CrossRef]
10. Yoshida, M.; Kikutani, T.; Tsuga, K.; Utanohara, Y.; Hayashi, R.; Akagawa, Y. Decreased tongue pressure reflects symptom of dysphagia. *Dysphagia* **2006**, *21*, 61–65. [CrossRef]
11. Suzuki, H.; Ayukawa, Y.; Ueno, Y.; Atsuta, I.; Jinnouchi, A.; Koyano, K. Relationship between Maximum Tongue Pressure Value and Age, Occlusal Status, or Body Mass Index among the Community-Dwelling Elderly. *Medicina* **2020**, *56*, e623. [CrossRef] [PubMed]
12. Takeuchi, K.; Ozawa, Y.; Hasegawa, J.; Tsuda, T.; Karino, T.; Ueda, A.; Toyoda, K. Usability of maximum tongue pressure measurement in patients with dysphagia or dysarthria—Using a newly developed measurement device. *Jpn. J. Dysphagia Rehabil.* **2012**, *16*, 165–174.
13. Persson, E.; Wårdh, I.; Östberg, P. Repetitive saliva swallowing test: Norms, clinical relevance and the impact of saliva secretion. *Dysphagia* **2019**, *34*, 271–278. [CrossRef]
14. Ichibayashi, R.; Honda, M.; Sekiya, H.; Yokomuro, H.; Yoshihara, K.; Urita, Y. Maximum tongue pressure as a measure of post-extubation swallowing ability. *Toho J. Med.* **2017**, *3*, 75–83.
15. Kanda, Y. Investigation of the Freely Available Easy-to-Use Software "EZR" for Medical Statistics. *Bone Marrow Transplant.* **2013**, *48*, 452–458. [CrossRef]
16. Rassameehiran, S.; Klomjit, S.; Mankongpaisarnrung, C.; Rakvit, A. Post-extubation Dysphagia. *Proc. Bayl Univ. Med. Cent.* **2015**, *28*, 18–20. [CrossRef]
17. El Solh, A.; Okada, M.; Bhat, A.; Pletrantoni, C. Swallowing disorders post orotracheal intubation in the elderly. *Intensive Care Med.* **2003**, *29*, 1451–1455. [CrossRef]
18. Epstein, S.K.; Ciubotaru, R.L. Independent effects of etiology of failure and time to reintubation on outcome for patients failing extubation. *Am. J. Respir. Crit. Care Med.* **1998**, *158*, 489–493. [CrossRef]
19. Mehta, S.; Nelson, D.L.; Klinger, J.R.; Buczko, G.B.; Levy, M.M. Prediction of post-extubation work of breathing. *Crit. Care Med.* **2000**, *28*, 1341–1346. [CrossRef]

20. Laghi, F.; D'Alfonso, N.; Tobin, M.J. Pattern of recovery from diaphragmatic fatigue over 24 hours. *J. Appl. Physiol.* **1995**, *79*, 539–546. [CrossRef]
21. Tsai, M.H.; Ku, S.C.; Wang, T.G.; Hsiao, T.Y.; Lee, J.J.; Chan, D.C.; Huang, G.H.; Chen, C.C. Swallowing dysfunction following endotracheal intubation. *Medicine* **2016**, *95*, e3871. [CrossRef] [PubMed]
22. de Larminat, V.; Montravers, P.; Dureuil, B.; Desmonts, J.M. Alteration in swallowing reflex after extubation in intensive care unit patients. *Crit. Care Med.* **1995**, *23*, 486–490. [CrossRef] [PubMed]
23. Can, B.; Ismagulova, N.; Enver, N.; Tufan, A.; Cinel, İ. Sarcopenic dysphagia following COVID-19 infection: A new danger. *Nutr. Clin. Pract.* **2021**, *36*, 828–832. [CrossRef] [PubMed]

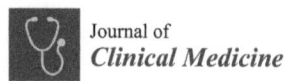

Article

Physical Inactivity and Sedentarism during and after Admission with Community-Acquired Pneumonia and the Risk of Readmission and Mortality: A Prospective Cohort Study

Camilla Koch Ryrsø [1,2,*], Arnold Matovu Dungu [1], Maria Hein Hegelund [1], Daniel Faurholt-Jepsen [3], Bente Klarlund Pedersen [2], Christian Ritz [4], Birgitte Lindegaard [1,2,5,†] and Rikke Krogh-Madsen [2,6,†]

[1] Department of Pulmonary and Infectious Diseases, Copenhagen University Hospital—North Zealand, 3400 Hillerød, Denmark
[2] Centre for Physical Activity Research, Copenhagen University Hospital—Rigshospitalet, 2100 Copenhagen, Denmark
[3] Department of Infectious Diseases, Copenhagen University Hospital, Rigshospitalet, 2100 Copenhagen, Denmark
[4] National Institute of Public Health, University of Southern Denmark, 1455 Copenhagen, Denmark
[5] Department of Clinical Medicine, University of Copenhagen, 2200 Copenhagen, Denmark
[6] Department of Infectious Diseases, Copenhagen University Hospital, Hvidovre, 2650 Copenhagen, Denmark
* Correspondence: camilla.koch.ryrsoe.01@regionh.dk
† These authors contributed equally to this work.

Abstract: Background: Bed rest with limited physical activity is common during admission. The aim was to determine the association between daily step count and physical activity levels during and after admission with community-acquired pneumonia (CAP) and the risk of readmission and mortality. Methods: A prospective cohort study of 166 patients admitted with CAP. Step count and physical activity were assessed with accelerometers during and after admission and were categorised as sedentary, light, or moderate-vigorous physical activity. Linear regression was used to assess the association between step count and length of stay. Logistic regression was used to assess the association between step count, physical activity level, and risk of readmission and mortality. Results: Patients admitted with CAP were sedentary, light physically active, and moderate-to-vigorous physically active 96.4%, 2.6%, and 0.9% of their time, respectively, with 1356 steps/d. For every 500-step increase in daily step count on day 1, the length of stay was reduced by 6.6%. For every 500-step increase in daily step count during admission, in-hospital and 30-day mortality was reduced. Increased light and moderate-to-vigorous physical activity during admission were associated with reduced risk of in-hospital and 30-day mortality. After discharge, patients increased their daily step count to 2654 steps/d and spent more time performing light and moderate-to-vigorous physical activity. For every 500-step increase in daily step count after discharge, the risk of readmission was reduced. Higher moderate-to-vigorous physical activity after discharge was associated with a reduced risk of readmission. Conclusions: Increased physical activity during admission was associated with a reduced length of stay and risk of mortality, whereas increased physical activity after discharge was associated with a reduced risk of readmission in patients with CAP. Interventions focusing on increasing physical activity levels should be prioritised to improve the prognosis of patients admitted with CAP.

Keywords: community-acquired pneumonia; hospital admission; length of stay; mortality; readmission; physical activity

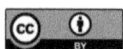

1. Introduction

Community-acquired pneumonia (CAP) remains a leading cause of hospital admission, with one in five patients being readmitted within 30 days after discharge [1,2]. Bed rest with limited physical activity is common during admission. In patients with CAP, both external (e.g., oxygen therapy, intravenous antibiotic treatment) and internal (e.g., fatigue, hypoxemia) factors limit physical activity during admission [3]. As a result, patients admitted with CAP spend over 90% of their in-hospital time being physically inactive, with 900–1300 steps/d during admission [4,5]. In comparison, the average number of daily steps is approximately 6500 steps/d for healthy individuals [6]. Physical inactivity is not only a concern among patients with low functional status; despite the ability to walk independently at admission, only 28% of medical patients admitted with respiratory, gastrointestinal, or renal disease walked during admission [7]. In patients with CAP, a lower daily step count during admission has been associated with a prolonged length of stay [4]. In addition, physical inactivity during admission has been associated with readmission and mortality in older medical patients admitted with respiratory, cardiovascular, or gastrointestinal diseases [8,9]. Hospital-associated deconditioning with loss of muscle mass and strength is a serious concern, as up to 40% of older patients lose the ability to perform activities of daily living after discharge [10–12]. For 40% of these patients, these newly acquired disabilities will never recover [12]. However, physical activity is a central and potentially modifiable factor to prevent hospital-associated functional decline and adverse outcomes in older medical patients [10,11]. In patients with CAP, an exercise intervention initiated during admission can, to some extent, counteract the negative consequences of physical inactivity on muscle strength and the ability to perform daily activities [13]. To our knowledge, no previous study has investigated the association between 24-h physical activity levels during and after admission on the prognosis in patients admitted with CAP.

We hypothesised that physical inactivity and sedentarism during admission and immediately after discharge were associated with an increased risk of severe outcomes in patients admitted with CAP. We aimed to determine 24-h physical activity levels and the daily step count during admission and immediately after discharge in patients with CAP and the association with prognosis, such as length of stay, 30-day readmission, and in-hospital and 30-day mortality.

2. Methods

2.1. Study Design, Settings, and Study Population

This study is part of the Surviving Pneumonia Cohort Study, a prospective cohort study including patients admitted with CAP at the Copenhagen University Hospital—North Zealand, Denmark. Inclusion criteria were age ≥ 18 years and suspected CAP defined as a new pulmonary infiltrate on chest X-ray or computed tomography scan and minimum 1 symptom consistent with CAP, e.g., fever ($\geq 38.0\ °C$), hypothermia ($<35.0\ °C$), cough, sputum production, pleuritic chest pain, dyspnea, or focal chest signs on auscultation. Exclusion criteria for the present study were no attachment of accelerometer at admission, paralysis of legs (non-ambulant), expected length of stay ≤ 48 h, or less than one day with ≤ 20 h physical activity data during admission. Patients were enrolled within the first 24 h of admission. Patients in the present study were included between January 2019 and April 2022.

2.2. Study Variables

Data were collected prospectively with standardised forms and were entered into a REDCap database. Information about demography, prior medical history, comorbidities, and clinical outcomes were collected during an interview at the study enrolment and from medical records. The CURB-65 score [14] was used to risk-stratify patients and was classified as mild (score 0–1), moderate (score 2), or severe (score 3–5) CAP. The combined burden of comorbidities was assessed by the Charlson Comorbidity Index [15] and categorised as 0, 1, or ≥ 2 comorbidities. Data upon admission to the intensive care unit (ICU), length of stay, readmission, and mortality were collected from medical records up to 30 days after discharge.

The self-reported physical activity level prior to admission was assessed with the short form of the international physical activity questionnaire (IPAQ) [16]. Patients were categorised into 3 levels of physical activity (low <600 metabolic equivalents of task (MET)-min/week, moderate ≥600 MET-min/week, or high ≥3000 MET-min/week) [17].

Physical activity levels were objectively assessed using the Axivity AX3 accelerometer. The accelerometers were initialised to measure at 100 Hz with ±8 g bandwidth using the Open Movement software (OmGui, version 1.0.0.43, Newcastle University, Newcastle upon Tyne, UK). The accelerometer was attached directly to the skin on the medial front of the right thigh, midway between the hip and knee joints, with its positive x-axis pointing inferiorly and its negative z-axis pointing anteriorly [18]. A 50 × 100 mm section of Mefix tape (Mölnlycke Health Care, Göteborg, Sweden) with a stripe of double-sided adhesive tape was placed on top of the clean, dry skin. The accelerometer was placed on the double-sided tape and secured to the site with a 110 × 140 mm piece of transparent film (Leukomed T, BNS medical GmbH, Hamburg, Germany). Patients were instructed to wear the accelerometer for up to 7 consecutive 24-h periods during admission or until discharge (if discharged before day 8) and 7 consecutive 24-h periods after discharge. Data were collected between 05:00 AM on day 1 and 05:00 AM on day 8.

Data from the accelerometers were downloaded in the original cwa file format using the OmGui software and converted to a binary gt3x compatible file format using a custom-made add-on to OmGui to assess intensity estimates using ActiLife (version 6.13.4, ActiGraph, Pensacola, FL, USA). The accelerometer wear time was determined manually using OmGui based on raw accelerometry. Data were extracted in 1 s epochs. Non-wear time was defined as ≥180 consecutive min of zero counts/min, allowing for up to 2 min of non-zero counts if the interruption was preceded or followed by ≥30 min of zero counts/min. A valid 24-h measurement was defined as at least 20 h of wear time. Patients were included if they had at least one day with ≥20 h out of 24 h of wear time [19]. Daily step counts were calculated from the step detection algorithm in ActiLife using the recordings of raw accelerations from the 3 axes [20]. Sedentary time was defined as time spent at ≤100 counts/min [21], light physical activity as 100–1951 counts/min, and moderate-to-vigorous physical activity as ≥1952 counts/min [22].

2.3. Outcomes

The primary outcome was a 30-day readmission, with secondary outcomes being length of stay and in-hospital and 30-day mortality. The days from discharge to readmission and cause of readmission were registered. Patients with multiple readmissions were registered with reference to the first readmission. All variables were collected from medical records. Age, sex, CURB-65, ICU admission, mechanical ventilation, non-invasive ventilation, and high flow therapy were viewed as potential confounders and were adjusted for. No stepwise selection process was applied.

2.4. Statistical Analysis

Data were described as counts (%) for categorical variables and either means (standard deviation (SD)) or medians (interquartile range (IQR)) for continuous variables as appropriate. Binary logistic regression analyses were used to assess the association between daily step count and physical activity levels (time spent in sedentary behaviour, light physical activity, and moderate-to-vigorous physical activity) and risk of 30-day readmission and in-hospital and 30-day mortality, respectively. Both unadjusted, univariate models and adjusted, multivariate models were fitted. To adjust for confounding, analyses included age, sex, CURB-65, ICU admission, mechanical ventilation, non-invasive ventilation, and high flow therapy. Linear regression was used to determine the association between step count on day 1 with the length of stay. Multivariate models included age, sex, and CURB-65. Model assumptions, including normality, were assessed using residual and quantile-quantile plots. Due to the skewed distribution of length of stay, the variable was log-transformed, and the regression coefficients were back-transformed to provide ratios.

Wilcoxon signed-rank tests were used to detect differences in daily step counts and physical activity levels from admission to after discharge. Chi-squared tests were used to explore differences in physical activity levels prior to admission between patients included before compared to during or after the COVID-19 lockdown. All p-values were two-sided, and significance levels were $p < 0.05$. Data were analysed using IBM SPSS Statistics version 25.

2.5. Research Ethics

Patients provided informed consent before enrolment. The study was approved by the Scientific Ethics Committee at the Capital Region of Denmark (H-18024256), registered on ClinicalTrials.gov (NCT03795662), and conducted according to the Declaration of Helsinki [23]. This reporting of the study followed the Strengthening the Reporting of Observational Studies in Epidemiology statement [24].

3. Results

Initially, 189 patients were included in the study; however, 23 patients were excluded from the analysis due to missing physical activity data from admission, leaving 166 patients with physical activity data during admission. After discharge, 89 patients were excluded from the analysis due to missing physical activity data, leaving 77 patients with physical activity data after discharge to be included in the analysis (Figure 1).

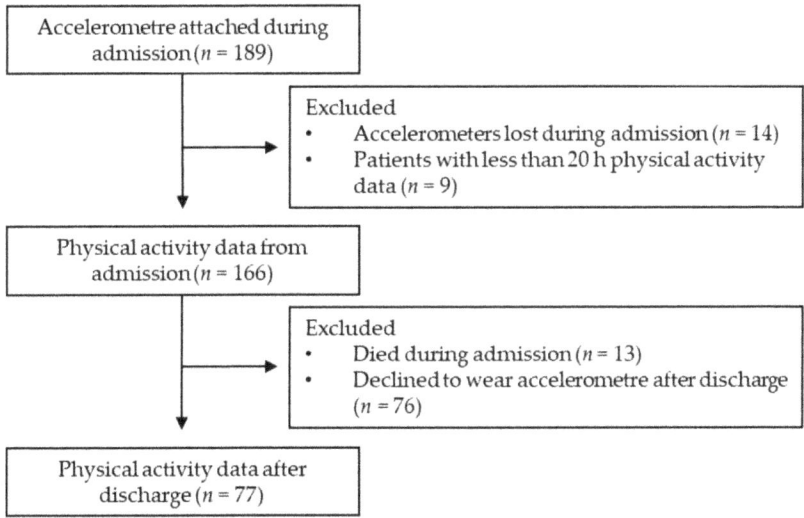

Figure 1. Flow chart of the study population.

3.1. Demography, Comorbidities, and Clinical Parameters

Patient characteristics are summarised in Table 1. The median age of the study population was 75 years, with 71.1% of the patients being 65 years of age or older. One hundred patients (60.2%) had ≥2 comorbidities, and 78 (50.3%) had mild CAP. Based on IPAQ, 80.1% of the patients had a low physical activity level prior to admission, while 13.2 and 6.6% had a moderate or high physical activity level (Table 1). There was no difference in physical activity levels prior to admission between patients included before the COVID-19 lockdown (January 2019–February 2020) and patients included during or after the COVID-19 lockdown (March 2020–April 2022, Supplementary Table S1).

Table 1. Baseline characteristics of 166 patients admitted with community-acquired pneumonia.

	Study Population (n = 166)
Age, median (IQR), years	75 (63–81)
Sex, male, n (%)	90 (54.2)
Charlson comorbidity index, median (IQR)	5 (3–6)
Number of comorbidities, n (%)	
0	24 (14.5)
1	42 (25.3)
≥2	100 (60.2)
Chronic obstructive pulmonary disease	62 (37.3)
Other chronic respiratory diseases	37 (22.3)
Malignancy	33 (19.9)
Diabetes	31 (18.7)
Chronic heart failure	30 (18.1)
Other chronic heart diseases	90 (54.2)
Cerebrovascular disease	26 (15.7)
Chronic kidney disease	7 (4.2)
Chronic liver disease	4 (2.4)
CURB-65	
0–1, n (%)	78 (50.3)
2, n (%)	57 (36.8)
3–5, n (%)	20 (12.9)
Physical activity level prior to admission	
Low, n (%)	121 (80.1)
Moderate, n (%)	20 (13.2)
High, n (%)	10 (6.6)
Clinical outcome	
Intravenous antibiotic treatment, n (%)	156 (94.0)
Oxygen therapy, n (%)	117 (70.5)
Intensive care unit, n (%)	5 (3.0)
Length of stay, median (IQR), days	7.2 (5.2–12.4)
In-hospital mortality, n (%)	13 (7.8)
30 days mortality, n (%)	16 (9.6)
30 days readmission, n (%)	37 (24.2)

CURB-65: confusion, urea, respiratory rate, blood pressure, and age ≥65 years. Missing variables: physical activity level (n = 15, 9.0%), CURB-65 (n = 11, 6.6%).

During admission, 156 patients (94.0%) received intravenous antibiotic treatment, and 117 (70.5%) were treated with supplementary oxygen. During admission, five patients (3.0%) were admitted to the ICU, and 13 (7.8%) died. Sixteen patients (9.6%) died within 30 days after discharge. The median length of stay was 7 days. Thirty-seven patients (24.2%) were readmitted within 30 days after discharge, with pulmonary conditions (e.g., CAP, acute exacerbation of chronic obstructive pulmonary disease (COPD)) being the most common causes of readmission (51.4%, Supplementary Table S2).

3.2. Physical Activity and Sedentary Behaviour during Admission and after Discharge

The mean wear time of the accelerometers was 4.0 ± 2.2 days during admission (45.4 ± 18.5% of admission time) and 6.3 ± 1.6 days after discharge (90.0 ± 22.4% of follow-up time). During admission, patients spent 96.4% of their time in sedentary behaviour, 2.6% in light physical activity, and 0.9% in moderate-to-vigorous physical activity. The median daily step count during admission was 1356 steps/d. After discharge, patients increased their daily step count to 2654 steps/d and spent more time in light and moderate-to-vigorous physical activity (4.2% and 1.8%, Table 2).

Table 2. Physical activity and sedentary behaviour during admission and after discharge among 77 patients admitted with community-acquired pneumonia.

	During Admission (n = 77)	After Discharge (n = 77)	p-Value
Time spent in sedentary behaviour, median (IQR), %	96.0 (94.8–96.9)	93.8 (91.8–95.7)	<0.001
Time spent in light physical activity, median (IQR), %	3.1 (2.2–3.9)	4.2 (2.9–6.1)	<0.001
Time spent in moderate-to-vigorous physical activity, median (IQR), %	1.0 (0.7–1.5)	1.8 (1.1–2.8)	<0.001
Steps, median (IQR), n/day	1588 (1130–2226)	2654 (1810–3847)	<0.001

Comparisons were made with Wilcoxon signed-rank tests.

3.3. Association between Physical Activity and Sedentary Behaviour during Admission and Prognosis

In a multivariable analysis adjusted for age, sex, and CURB-65, length of stay was reduced by 6.6% (95% CI 2.0–10.9%; $p < 0.01$) for every 500-step increase in daily step count on day 1. There was no association between daily step count or time spent in sedentary behaviour, light physical activity, and moderate-to-vigorous physical activity during admission and risk of 30-day readmission (Figure 2).

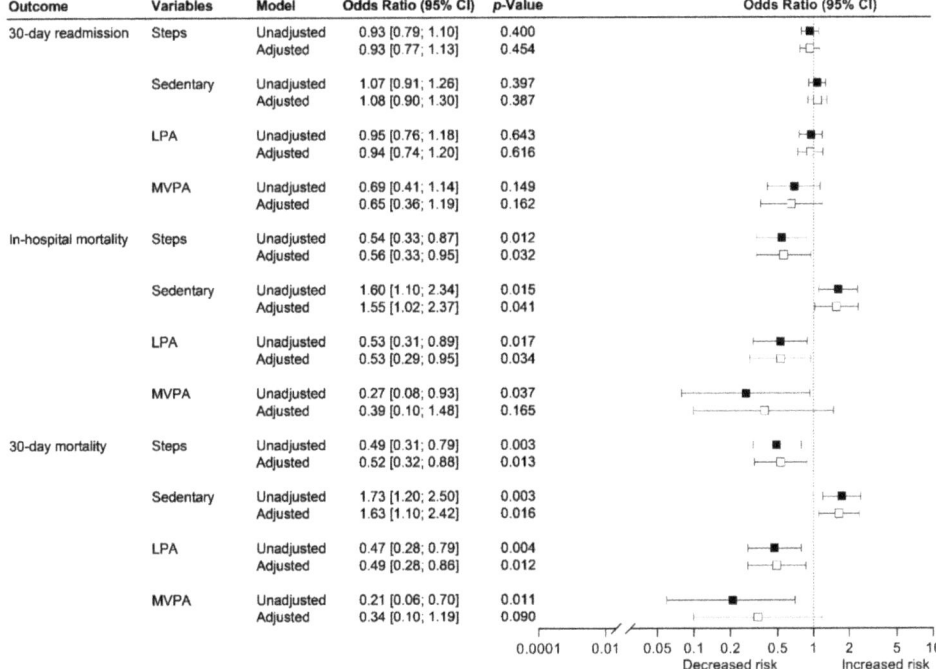

Figure 2. Association between physical activity and sedentary behaviour during admission and risk of readmission and mortality among 166 patients admitted with community-acquired pneumonia. The association between daily step count and physical activity level during admission and risk of 30-day readmission, in-hospital mortality, and 30-day mortality were analysed using unadjusted and adjusted logistic regression models (adjustments: age, sex, and CURB-65 (white)). Steps: Odds ratio per 500-step increase in daily step count during admission. The patients who died in the hospital are not included in the analyses for readmission. LPA: light physical activity, MVPA: moderate-to-vigorous physical activity.

Risk of in-hospital and 30-day mortality was reduced between 44–48% for every additional 500-step increase in daily step count during admission (Figure 2). Further adjustment with ICU admission, mechanical ventilation, non-invasive ventilation, and high flow therapy did not change the estimates, but models were no longer significant. Risk of in-hospital and 30-day mortality increased between 55–63% for every 1-percentage point increase in sedentary behaviour during admission, corresponding to a 14-min increase in sedentary behaviour (Figure 2). Further adjustment with ICU admission, mechanical ventilation, non-invasive ventilation, and high flow therapy did not change the estimates, but models were no longer significant.

Risk of in-hospital and 30-day mortality decreased between 47–51% for every 1-percentage point increase in light physical activity during admission (Figure 2). Further adjustment with ICU admission, mechanical ventilation, non-invasive ventilation, and high flow therapy did not change the estimates, but models were no longer significant.

Risk of in-hospital and 30-day mortality decreased between 73–79% for every 1-percentage point increase in moderate-to-vigorous physical activity during admission (Figure 2). Further adjustment with ICU admission, mechanical ventilation, non-invasive ventilation, and high flow therapy did not change the estimates, but models were no longer significant.

3.4. Association between Physical Activity and Sedentary Behaviour after Discharge and Prognosis

Risk of 30-day readmission was reduced between 21–24% for every additional 500-step increase in daily step count after discharge (Figure 3).

Outcome	Variables	Model	Odds Ratio (95% CI)	p-Value
30-day readmission	Steps	Unadjusted	0.79 [0.64; 0.97]	0.022
		Adjusted	0.76 [0.53; 0.98]	0.036
	Sedentary	Unadjusted	1.24 [1.02; 1.51]	0.029
		Adjusted	1.29 [1.01; 1.64]	0.039
	LPA	Unadjusted	0.81 [0.62; 1.04]	0.098
		Adjusted	0.82 [0.61; 1.10]	0.131
	MVPA	Unadjusted	0.46 [0.25; 0.85]	0.012
		Adjusted	0.37 [0.17; 0.84]	0.014
30-day mortality	Steps	Unadjusted	0.33 [0.10; 1.10]	0.071
		Adjusted	0.41 [0.12; 1.44]	0.166
	Sedentary	Unadjusted	2.55 [0.99; 6.56]	0.052
		Adjusted	1.99 [0.74; 5.35]	0.174
	LPA	Unadjusted	0.29 [0.08; 1.06]	0.061
		Adjusted	0.44 [0.11; 1.73]	0.241
	MVPA	Unadjusted	0.01 [0.00; 1.38]	0.068
		Adjusted	0.05 [0.00; 4.17]	0.182

Figure 3. Association between physical activity and sedentary behaviour after discharge and risk of readmission and mortality among 77 patients admitted with community-acquired pneumonia. The association between daily step count and physical activity level after discharge and risk of 30-day readmission and mortality were analysed using unadjusted (black) and adjusted logistic regression models (adjustments: age, sex, and CURB-65 (white)). Steps: Odds ratio per 500-step increase in daily step count after discharge. LPA: light physical activity, MVPA: moderate-to-vigorous physical activity.

Risk of 30-day readmission increased by 24–29% for every 1-percentage point increase in sedentary behaviour after discharge (Figure 3). There was no association between time spent in light physical activity and risk of 30-day readmission.

Risk of 30-day readmission decreased by 54–63% for every 1-percentage point increase in moderate-to-vigorous physical activity after discharge (Figure 3).

There was no association between daily step count or time spent in sedentary behaviour, light physical activity, and moderate-to-vigorous physical activity after discharge and risk of 30-day mortality (Figure 3).

4. Discussion

We examined the impact of physical activity levels during admission and immediately after discharge on the prognosis in patients with CAP. Overall, patients admitted with CAP spend most of their time in sedentary behaviour with a low daily step count. After discharge, patients increase their daily step count and engage in more light and moderate-to-vigorous physical activity. First, our results showed that increased daily step count on the first day of admission is associated with a reduced length of stay. Second, increased physical activity and less time spent in sedentary behaviour during admission are associated with a reduced risk of in-hospital and 30-day mortality. Third, increased physical activity and less time spent in sedentary behaviour after discharge are associated with a reduced risk of 30-day readmission. Finally, our findings demonstrate the crucial association between physical activity during admission and immediately after discharge on prognosis in patients with CAP.

Bed rest with limited physical activity is common during admission. Patients admitted with CAP spent over 96% of their in-hospital time in sedentary behaviour, with only 1356 steps/d, which is similar to previous observations [4,5]. Further, we showed that, for every 500-step increase in daily step count on the first day of admission, the length of stay was reduced by 6.6%, corresponding to 0.5 days reduction. Our findings are consistent with a recent study by Rice and colleagues [4] showing an 11% reduced length of stay, corresponding to 0.4 days reduction, for every 500-step increase in daily step count during admission in patients with CAP.

An increased daily step count during admission was associated with a 44–51% reduced risk of in-hospital and 30-day mortality. In comparison, a previous study of older medical patients admitted with respiratory, cardiovascular, or gastrointestinal diseases showed a 2% reduced risk of 2-year mortality with an increased daily step count in the first 24 h of admission [9]. Similarly, a decline in daily step count from the first to the last 24 h of admission was associated with a 4-fold increased risk of 2-year mortality [9]. Further, we showed that an increase in light physical activity and a concurrent reduction in sedentarism during admission was associated with a 47–53% reduced risk of in-hospital and 30-day mortality. While physical activity is associated with an improved prognosis, an important issue to address is whether the low physical activity levels seen in patients admitted with CAP are simply a marker of disease severity, where severely ill patients are predominantly sedentary, and thus their poor disease outcomes should be attributed to their disease severity alone rather than a combination of disease severity and sedentarism. In a secondary analysis of the association between physical activity during admission and mortality, we included multiple variables (ICU admission, mechanical ventilation, non-invasive ventilation, and high flow therapy) to control for disease severity. After these adjustments, the estimates for the association between physical activity during admission and risk of in-hospital and 30-day mortality remained the same, but models were no longer significant.

We did not find any association between daily step count during admission and risk of 30-day readmission, which is in line with earlier observations from patients with CAP [4]. However, a 10% reduced risk of 30-day readmission has previously been reported in older medical patients admitted with respiratory, cardiovascular, or gastrointestinal diseases with an increased daily step count during admission [8].

Similar to previous studies measuring physical activity levels in patients admitted with CAP, we included patients aged ≥18 years [4,5]. Though the risk of CAP-requiring admissions increases with age, younger patients (≤64 years) admitted with CAP are often characterised with multiple comorbidities, which increases the risk of disease severity leading to prolonged length of stay and bed rest [25]. Even though earlier bed rest studies have shown that older healthy individuals are more susceptible to loss of muscle than younger during short-term bed rest [26], a substantial loss of muscle mass and strength still occurs in younger individuals [27,28].

Physical inactivity is not only a concern during admission but proceeds long after discharge. In the week following discharge, the daily step count significantly increased to 2654 steps/d, which is similar to previous observations from patients with CAP [5]. Further, we showed that increased daily step count and moderate-to-vigorous physical activity after discharge were associated with a 21–63% reduced risk of 30-day readmission in patients with CAP. Similarly, in a study of older medical patients admitted with respiratory, cardiovascular, or gastrointestinal diseases, increased daily step count the week following discharge was associated with a 15% reduced risk of 30-day readmission [29].

We did not find any association between the physical activity level after discharge and risk of 30-day mortality, as only 2 out of 77 patients died during the 30-day follow-up period from discharge. However, we still believe it is important to report odds ratios and confidence intervals to provide a quantification of the magnitude of the association. Results from our study could indicate that physical activity during admission is more related to survival, whereas physical activity after discharge is associated with recovery after discharge and whether readmissions can be prevented. Although physical inactivity often reflects disease severity, encouraging physical activity in all disease stages could be a powerful strategy to reduce the risk of readmission.

After discharge, the patients spent less time in sedentary behaviour than during admission, which is in line with observations from previous studies of patients with CAP [5,30]. However, in contrast to a study by Clausen and colleagues [5] of patients admitted with CAP, patients in our study spent considerably more time in sedentary behaviour after discharge (20.2 h/d vs 22.5 h/d). Differences in inclusion criteria between the studies could explain the different findings, as Clausen and colleagues [5] excluded patients who were admitted to the ICU within 24 h of admission. In contrast, we included patients despite ICU admission. Indeed, patients admitted to the ICU might display more sedentarism and delayed increase in physical activity level after discharge as a consequence of critical illness [31]. Our results could suggest that promoting physical activity through intervention may be required to increase physical activity levels during admission and after discharge. However, randomised controlled trials comparing the effect of standard of care combined with exercise training to standard of care alone are needed to explore whether an increased physical activity level during admission and after discharge improves the prognosis among patients with CAP.

Our findings emphasise the powerful association between the prognosis and interruption of sedentarism with increased physical activity levels in patients with CAP both during admission and immediately after discharge. It is, however, not known if low physical activity is a marker or a cause of severe disease. Nonetheless, hospitals play a crucial role in providing opportunities for patients to be physically active despite disease stages and acute illness. The prescription of exercise as a standardised part of the treatment for CAP could motivate patients to be more physically active even after discharge from the hospital. Indeed, previous studies of patients with CAP have shown that early and progressive mobilisation initiated within the first 24 h of admission reduces the length of stay by 1.1 to 2.1 days without increasing the risk of adverse events [32,33]. However, no study has to date looked at the effects of exercise training initiated during admission on the prognosis in patients with CAP.

Nonetheless, exercise training initiated immediately after discharge in patients admitted with acute exacerbation of COPD has been shown to reduce the number of days in the hospital and the risk of readmission and mortality [34]. These previous findings suggest that increasing physical activity levels through exercise interventions could be a way to improve the prognosis of patients admitted with CAP. Further results from our study suggest that relatively small increases in physical activity levels, both during admission and immediately after discharge, are associated with significant improvements in the prognosis of patients with CAP.

Strength and Limitations

The strength of this study is the large sample size, the broad inclusion criteria (i.e., including severely ill patients admitted to the ICU and patients who used walking aids), the use of validated accelerometers to assess physical activity both during admission and after discharge, and the large number of activity hours recorded (15,741 h during admission and 11,640 h after discharge). Further, we add to the current evidence by showing low physical activity levels in patients admitted with CAP. However, this is the first study showing the association between low physical activity levels and the increased risk of readmission and mortality in patients with CAP.

Our study had some limitations. First, there is a risk of selection and inclusion bias, as informed consent had to be obtained within the first 24 h of admission. Therefore, we cannot rule out that patients' refusal to participate in our study could be associated with the severity of their disease. Second, we excluded patients with a length of stay $\leq$48 h and $\leq$20 h of valid physical activity measurement. This might have led to the exclusion of patients with higher physical activity levels and less disease severity. However, we measured patients as many days as logistically possible and only included patients in the analysis if they had at least 1 day with $\geq$20 h out of 24 h of wear time to ensure both day and night measurement. Third, we only had physical activity data after discharge from 77 out of the 153 patients who were discharged alive, as patients refused to wear the accelerometer after discharge. However, there were no differences in age, sex, Charlson comorbidity index, number of comorbidities, CURB-65, or physical activity levels during admission between patients who wore an accelerometer after discharge and those who refused to wear it. Therefore, we assume that the 77 patients who wore the accelerometer after discharge are representative of the whole study population.

5. Conclusions

The present study provides evidence that physical inactivity and sedentarism are correlated with prolonged length of stay and increased risk of readmission and mortality in patients admitted with CAP. However, randomised controlled trials are needed to establish whether exercise training initiated during admission improves prognosis among patients with CAP.

Supplementary Materials: The following supporting information can be downloaded at: https://www.mdpi.com/article/10.3390/jcm11195923/s1, Table S1: Physical activity level prior to admission between patients included before the COVID-19 lockdown compared to patients included during or after the lockdown; Table S2: Cause of 30-day readmission.

Author Contributions: C.K.R., B.L., D.F.-J. and R.K.-M. conceptualised the study. C.K.R., A.M.D. and M.H.H. led the data acquisition. C.K.R. verified the underlying data and analysed it. C.K.R., B.L., D.F.-J., B.K.P., C.R. and R.K.-M. led the data interpretation. C.K.R. drafted the manuscript. All authors critically revised the manuscript for important intellectual content, approved the final version, and are accountable for all aspects of the work presented. All authors designated as authors qualify for authorship and those who qualify for authorship are listed. All authors have read and agreed to the published version of the manuscript.

Funding: The study was supported by grants from the Research Council at Copenhagen University Hospital—North Zealand, Denmark (funding number: none), and Grosserer L.F. Foght Foundation (funding number: none). The Centre for Physical Activity Research (CFAS) is supported by Tryg-Fonden (grants ID 101390, ID 20045, and ID 125132). The funding source was not involved in the study design, data collection, data analysis, interpretation of data, writing of the paper, or decision to submit the report for publication.

Institutional Review Board Statement: The study was conducted according to the guidelines of the Declaration of Helsinki and approved by the Scientific Ethics Committee at the Capital Region of Denmark (H-18024256). The study was registered on ClinicalTrials.gov (NCT03795662).

Informed Consent Statement: Informed consent was obtained from all patients before enrolment.

Data Availability Statement: Datasets used for the current study are not publicly available. However, relevant pseudonymised data can be accessed upon a reasonable request to the corresponding author. The lead author affirms that the manuscript is an honest, accurate, and transparent account of the study being reported; that no important aspects of the study have been omitted; and that any discrepancies from the study as planned have been explained.

Acknowledgments: The research nurses Malene Pilegaard Schønnemann, Hanne Hallager, and Christina Brix are acknowledged for their technical assistance. National Institute of Public Health, University of Southern Denmark, and TrygFonden are acknowledged for lending the applied accelerometers.

Conflicts of Interest: All authors have completed the ICMJE uniform disclosure form and declare support from the Research Council at Copenhagen University Hospital—North Zealand, Denmark, and Grosserer L.F. Foght Foundation for the submitted work; no financial relationships with any organisations that might have an interest in the submitted work in the previous years; no other relationships or activities that could appear to have influenced the submitted work.

Abbreviations

CAP: community-acquired pneumonia; CI: confidence interval; COPD: chronic obstructive pulmonary disease; CMP: counts per min; CURB-65: confusion, urea, respiratory rate, blood pressure, age ≥ 65 years; ICU: intensive care unit; IPAQ: international physical activity questionnaire; IQR: interquartile range; LPA: light physical activity; MVPA: moderate-to-vigorous physical activity; OR: odds ratio; SD: standard deviation.

References

1. Lozano, R.; Naghavi, M.; Foreman, K.; Lim, S.; Shibuya, K.; Aboyans, V.; Abraham, J.; Adair, T.; Aggarwal, R.; Ahn, S.Y.; et al. Global and regional mortality from 235 causes of death for 20 age groups in 1990 and 2010: A systematic analysis for the Global Burden of Disease Study 2010. *Lancet* **2012**, *380*, 2095–2128. [CrossRef]
2. Petersen, P.T.; Egelund, G.B.; Jensen, A.V.; Andersen, S.B.; Pedersen, M.F.; Rohde, G.; Ravn, P. Associations between biomarkers at discharge and comorbidities and risk of readmission after community-acquired pneumonia: A retrospective cohort study. *Eur. J. Clin. Microbiol.* **2018**, *37*, 1103–1111. [CrossRef] [PubMed]
3. Kawamura, K.; Kato, T.; Sakai, H.; Setaka, Y.; Hirose, Y.; Oozone, K.; Aita, I.; Tomita, K. Investigation into the mobility of elderly patients with pneumonia using triaxial accelerometer data. *Phys. Ther. Res.* **2019**, *22*, 73–80. [CrossRef] [PubMed]
4. Rice, H.; Hill, K.; Fowler, R.; Watson, C.; Waterer, G.; Harrold, M. Reduced Step Count and Clinical Frailty in Hospitalized Adults With Community-Acquired Pneumonia. *Respir. Care* **2020**, *65*, 455–463. [CrossRef] [PubMed]
5. Clausen, L.N.; Børgesen, M.; Ravn, P.; Møller, T. Fast-track pneumonia pathway focusing on early progressive mobilisation: A clinical feasibility study. *ERJ Open Res.* **2019**, *5*, 00012-2019. [CrossRef]
6. Paluch, A.E.; Bajpai, S.; Bassett, D.R.; Carnethon, M.R.; Ekelund, U.; Evenson, K.R.; Galuska, D.A.; Jefferis, B.J.; Kraus, W.E.; Lee, I.-M.; et al. Daily steps and all-cause mortality: A meta-analysis of 15 international cohorts. *Lancet Public Health* **2022**, *7*, e219–e228. [CrossRef]
7. Callen, B.L.; Mahoney, J.E.; Grieves, C.B.; Wells, T.J.; Enloe, M. Frequency of hallway ambulation by hospitalized older adults on medical units of an academic hospital. *Geriatr. Nurs.* **2004**, *25*, 212–217. [CrossRef]
8. Fisher, S.R.; Graham, J.E.; Ottenbacher, K.J.; Deer, R.; Ostir, G.V. Inpatient Walking Activity to Predict Readmission in Older Adults. *Arch. Phys. Med Rehabil.* **2016**, *97* (Suppl. S9), S226–S231. [CrossRef]
9. Ostir, G.V.; Berges, I.M.; Kuo, Y.-F.; Goodwin, J.S.; Fisher, S.R.; Guralnik, J.M. Mobility activity and its value as a prognostic indicator of survival in hospitalized older adults. *J. Am. Geriatr. Soc.* **2013**, *61*, 551–557. [CrossRef]
10. Zisberg, A.; Shadmi, E.; Gur-Yaish, N.; Tonkikh, O.; Sinoff, G. Hospital-associated functional decline: The role of hospitalization processes beyond individual risk factors. *J. Am. Geriatr. Soc.* **2015**, *63*, 55–62. [CrossRef]
11. Agmon, M.; Zisberg, A.; Gil, E.; Rand, D.; Gur-Yaish, N.; Azriel, M. Association Between 900 Steps a Day and Functional Decline in Older Hospitalized Patients. *JAMA Intern. Med.* **2017**, *177*, 272–274. [CrossRef] [PubMed]
12. Sager, M.A.; Franke, T.; Inouye, S.K.; Landefeld, C.S.; Morgan, T.M.; Rudberg, M.A.; Siebens, H.; Winograd, C.H. Functional Outcomes of Acute Medical Illness and Hospitalization in Older Persons. *Arch. Intern. Med.* **1996**, *156*, 645–652. [CrossRef] [PubMed]
13. José, A.; Corso, S.D. Inpatient rehabilitation improves functional capacity, peripheral muscle strength and quality of life in patients with community-acquired pneumonia: A randomised trial. *J. Physiother.* **2016**, *62*, 96–102. [CrossRef] [PubMed]
14. Lim, W.S.; Van Der Eerden, M.M.; Laing, R.; Boersma, W.G.; Karalus, N.; Town, G.I.; Lewis, S.A.; Macfarlane, J.T. Defining community acquired pneumonia severity on presentation to hospital: An international derivation and validation study. *Thorax* **2003**, *58*, 377–382. [CrossRef] [PubMed]

15. Charlson, M.E.; Pompei, P.; Ales, K.L.; MacKenzie, C.R. A new method of classifying prognostic comorbidity in longitudinal studies: Development and validation. *J. Chronic Dis.* **1987**, *40*, 373–383. [CrossRef]
16. Hagströmer, M.; Oja, P.; Sjöström, M. The International Physical Activity Questionnaire (IPAQ): A study of concurrent and construct validity. *Public Health Nutr.* **2006**, *9*, 755–762. [CrossRef]
17. International Physical Activity Questionnaire. *Guidelines for the Data Processing and Analysis of the International Physical Activity Questionnaire (IPAQ)—Short Form*; version 2.0, The IPAQ group. 2004.
18. Schneller, M.B.; Bentsen, P.; Nielsen, G.; Brønd, J.C.; Ried-Larsen, M.; Mygind, E.; Schipperijn, J. Measuring Children's Physical Activity: Compliance Using Skin-Taped Accelerometers. *Med. Sci. Sports Exerc.* **2017**, *49*, 1261–1269. [CrossRef]
19. Chim, H.Q. Physical Activity Behavior and Learning in Higher Education. Ph.D. Thesis, Maastricht University, Maastricht, The Netherlands, 2021.
20. Stenbäck, V.; Leppäluoto, J.; Leskelä, N.; Viitala, L.; Vihriälä, E.; Gagnon, D.; Tulppo, M.; Herzig, K.-H. Step detection and energy expenditure at different speeds by three accelerometers in a controlled environment. *Sci. Rep.* **2021**, *11*, 20005. [CrossRef]
21. Wong, S.L.; Colley, R.; Gorber, S.C.; Tremblay, M. Actical accelerometer sedentary activity thresholds for adults. *J. Phys. Act. Health* **2011**, *8*, 587–591. [CrossRef]
22. Freedson, P.S.; Melanson, E.; Sirard, J. Calibration of the Computer Science and Applications, Inc. accelerometer. *Med. Sci. Sports Exerc.* **1998**, *30*, 777–781. [CrossRef]
23. World Medical Association. World Medical Association Declaration of Helsinki: Ethical Principles for Medical Research Involving Human Subjects. *JAMA* **2013**, *310*, 2191–2194. [CrossRef] [PubMed]
24. von Elm, E.; Altman, D.G.; Egger, M.; Pocock, S.J.; Gøtzsche, P.C.; Vandenbroucke, J.P.; STROBE Initiative. The Strengthening the Reporting of Observational Studies in Epidemiology (STROBE) statement: Guidelines for reporting observational studies. *J. Clin. Epidemiol.* **2008**, *61*, 344–349. [CrossRef] [PubMed]
25. Ruiz, L.A.; España, P.P.; Gómez, A.; Bilbao, A.; Jaca, C.; Arámburu, A.; Capelastegui, A.; Restrepo, M.I.; Zalacain, R. Age-related differences in management and outcomes in hospitalised healthy and well-functioning bacteremic pneumococcal pneumonia patients: A cohort study. *BMC Geriatr.* **2017**, *17*, 130. [CrossRef] [PubMed]
26. Tanner, R.E.; Brunker, L.B.; Agergaard, J.; Barrows, K.M.; Briggs, R.A.; Kwon, O.S.; Young, L.M.; Hopkins, P.N.; Volpi, E.; Marcus, R.; et al. Age-related differences in lean mass, protein synthesis and skeletal muscle markers of proteolysis after bed rest and exercise rehabilitation. *J. Physiol.* **2015**, *593*, 4259–4273. [CrossRef] [PubMed]
27. Krogh-Madsen, R.; Thyfault, J.P.; Broholm, C.; Mortensen, O.H.; Olsen, R.H.; Mounier, R.; Plomgaard, P.; van Hall, G.; Booth, F.W.; Pedersen, B.K. A 2-wk reduction of ambulatory activity attenuates peripheral insulin sensitivity. *J. Appl. Physiol.* **2010**, *108*, 1034–1040. [CrossRef] [PubMed]
28. Nielsen, S.T.; Harder-Lauridsen, N.M.; Benatti, F.B.; Wedell-Neergaard, A.-S.; Lyngbæk, M.P.; Moller, K.; Pedersen, B.K.; Krogh-Madsen, R. The effect of 8 days of strict bed rest on the incretin effect in healthy volunteers. *J. Appl. Physiol.* **2016**, *120*, 608–614. [CrossRef] [PubMed]
29. Fisher, S.R.; Kuo, Y.-F.; Sharma, G.; Raji, M.A.; Kumar, A.; Goodwin, J.S.; Ostir, G.V.; Ottenbacher, K.J. Mobility after hospital discharge as a marker for 30-day readmission. *J. Gerontol. A Biol. Sci. Med. Sci.* **2013**, *68*, 805–810. [CrossRef]
30. Jawad, B.N.; Petersen, J.; Andersen, O.; Pedersen, M.M. Variations in physical activity and sedentary behavior during and after hospitalization in acutely admitted older medical patients: A longitudinal study. *BMC Geriatr.* **2022**, *22*, 209. [CrossRef]
31. Borges, R.C.; Carvalho, C.R.F.; Colombo, A.S.; Borges, M.P.d.S.; Soriano, F.G. Physical activity, muscle strength, and exercise capacity 3 months after severe sepsis and septic shock. *Intensive Care Med.* **2015**, *41*, 1433–1444. [CrossRef]
32. Carratalà, J.; Garcia-Vidal, C.; Ortega, L.; Fernández-Sabé, N.; Clemente, M.; Albero, G.; López, M.; Castellsagué, X.; Dorca, J.; Verdaguer, R.; et al. Effect of a 3-step critical pathway to reduce duration of intravenous antibiotic therapy and length of stay in community-acquired pneumonia: A randomized controlled trial. *Arch. Intern. Med.* **2012**, *172*, 922–928. [CrossRef]
33. Mundy, L.M.; Leet, T.L.; Darst, K.; Schnitzler, M.A.; Dunagan, W.C. Early mobilization of patients hospitalized with community-acquired pneumonia. *Chest* **2003**, *124*, 883–889. [CrossRef] [PubMed]
34. Ryrsø, C.K.; Godtfredsen, N.S.; Kofod, L.M.; Lavesen, M.; Mogensen, L.; Tobberup, R.; Farver-Vestergaard, I.; Callesen, H.E.; Tendal, B.; Lange, P.; et al. Lower mortality after early supervised pulmonary rehabilitation following COPD-exacerbations: A systematic review and meta-analysis. *BMC Pulm. Med.* **2018**, *18*, 154. [CrossRef] [PubMed]

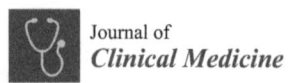

Article

A Paradigm Shift in the Diagnosis of Aspiration Pneumonia in Older Adults

Yuki Yoshimatsu [1,2,*] and David G. Smithard [1,2]

[1] Elderly Care, Queen Elizabeth Hospital, Lewisham and Greenwich NHS Trust, London SE18 4QH, UK
[2] Centre for Exercise Activity and Rehabilitation, School of Human Sciences, University of Greenwich, London SE10 9LS, UK
* Correspondence: yukitsukihana0105@gmail.com

Abstract: In older adults, community-acquired pneumonia (CAP) is often aspiration-related. However, as aspiration pneumonia (AP) lacks clear diagnostic criteria, the reported prevalence and clinical management vary greatly. We investigated what clinical factors appeared to influence the diagnosis of AP and non-AP in a clinical setting and reconsidered a more clinically relevant approach. Medical records of patients aged ≥75 years admitted with CAP were reviewed retrospectively. A total of 803 patients (134 APs and 669 non-APs) were included. The AP group had significantly higher rates of frailty, had higher SARC-F scores, resided in institutions, had neurologic conditions, previous pneumonia diagnoses, known dysphagia, and were more likely to present with vomiting or coughing on food. Nil by mouth orders, speech therapist referrals, and broad-spectrum antibiotics were significantly more common, while computed tomography scans and blood cultures were rarely performed; alternative diagnoses, such as cancer and pulmonary embolism, were detected significantly less. AP is diagnosed more commonly in frail patients, while aspiration is the underlying aetiology in most types of pneumonia. A presumptive diagnosis of AP may deny patients necessary investigation and management. We suggest a paradigm shift in the way we approach older patients with CAP; rather than trying to differentiate AP and non-AP, it would be more clinically relevant to recognise all pneumonia as just pneumonia, and assess their swallowing functions, causative organisms, and investigate alternative diagnoses or underlying causes of dysphagia. This will enable appropriate clinical management.

Keywords: dysphagia; swallowing disorder; aspiration; diagnosis; differential; community-acquired pneumonia; CAP; frailty

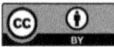

1. Introduction

In this unprecedented ageing world, clinicians are facing the increasing impacts of community-acquired pneumonia (CAP) in older adults on a regular basis. Its high prevalence and morbidity are causing large medical burdens, while also imposing socioeconomic consequences on the whole of society [1]. The incidence of pneumonia has increased from 1.5 to 2.2 per 1000 person years between 2002 and 2017 [2], with the prevalence being 6 times higher in those aged ≥75 years old compared to those <60 years of age [3]. CAP has a mortality of 2–5/1000 years [4,5], and in 2019 there were 2.5 million deaths from pneumonia [6].

Aspiration is considered to be the likely aetiology of pneumonia in up to 90% of older adults [7], where dysphagia is common [8]. Consequently, nearly all pneumonia will be associated with the aspiration of oropharyngeal secretions. However, swallowing problems alone may not be the cause of aspiration pneumonia (AP) [9], and the clinical effects may depend on the frailty of the patient, the oral microbiome load due to insufficient oral care, and a decompensated airway clearance [10,11]. Having an adequate cough reflex, the urge to cough, and the necessary pulmonary function are all important aspects in the prevention of pneumonia. Sarcopenia is also known to be a risk factor for pneumonia in older people [12]. Many people will have a pre-existing compromised swallow, a previously unidentified swallowing problem, or a decompensated swallow due to illness and frailty. Patients with a diagnosis of AP are at risk of longer and more frequent admissions, are more likely to be frail, and have multiple comorbidities [13,14]. Therefore, their clinical management requires multi-professional assessment and care, in addition to those for CAP in general.

There are no clear diagnostic criteria for AP, and the diagnosis is often presumptive [7]. British and American pneumonia guidelines do not state a definition [15,16]; Japanese guidelines merely state a list of risk factors for aspiration and pneumonia, explaining that clear criteria cannot be easily established [17]. Understandably, this implies an inconsistency in what clinicians and researchers infer when they mention the term "AP". Its reported ratio also varies greatly, ranging from 5.6% to as high as 90% among those diagnosed with CAP [7,13,18–20]. A need for clarity in the diagnosis of AP has been voiced for decades. Though some researchers have made suggestions [21], there are yet to be unified criteria.

Subsequent to the absence of a unified definition of AP, the management of pneumonia in older adults remains variable [22]. When a diagnosis of AP is made, it is common to restrict patients' oral intake. When a patient has a repetitive diagnosis of AP, it leads clinicians to suspect entry of food and liquids into the airway as being the cause, and often to the decision of nil by mouth (NBM), while the need for (artificial) nutrition is ignored. However, how can clinicians make such crucial decisions based on such unreliable diagnoses? With the prognosis of AP being poor [22], adequate management is crucial.

Though there have been increasing numbers of studies suggesting how a diagnosis of AP is reached [21,23], the appropriateness of the diagnosis or how AP is actually being diagnosed in the daily clinical setting remains largely unexplored. This is especially so in the UK, as many studies originate from Japan, Spain, and elsewhere [23]. Without real-world data, it is impossible to know the real issues that need to be addressed. Therefore, we designed a study to investigate what clinical factors appear to influence the diagnosis of AP, and how the differentiation affects its management in the acute geriatric setting. This study was performed to reconsider a clinically relevant way to diagnose AP in older adults.

2. Materials and Methods

2.1. Study Design

This was a retrospective cohort study analysing how older patients admitted with CAP were diagnosed as having AP or non-AP, and whether their management differed depending on the diagnosis. The study was performed at Queen Elizabeth Hospital (Lewisham and Greenwich NHS Trust), a local 521-bed acute care hospital serving the south-eastern London area of England. Ethical approval was provided by the Lewisham and Greenwich NHS Trust as instituted by the Declaration of Helsinki, and informed consent was waived.

2.2. Patients

Patients aged ≥75 years admitted with a diagnosis of CAP from the emergency department from 1 January to 31 December, 2021 were included in the study. A list of patients with pneumonia or pneumonitis as a primary or secondary diagnosis of admission was obtained from the hospital database. Exclusion criteria were admissions for hospital-acquired pneumonia (HAP), cases that were diagnosed with pneumonia after initially being admitted for a different condition, COVID-19 pneumonitis, and cases without pneumonia according to medical records (a discrepancy between the coded database and written medical records). Patients diagnosed with infectious exacerbation of chronic obstructive pulmonary disease (COPD) were included if they were also diagnosed with pneumonia. Patients who were admitted multiple times during the study period were only included for the first admission, and any admissions thereafter were excluded.

2.3. Definitions

CAP was defined as pneumonia developing in the community or within 48 h of hospital admission [15], and HAP was defined as pneumonia not incubating at the time of hospital admission and occurring 48 h or more after admission [24], according to the American Thoracic Society (ATS) and the Infectious Diseases Society of America (IDSA) guidelines. The diagnoses of pneumonia and AP were extracted according to what was documented on the consultant physician ward round at the time of admission. This was because our study intended to investigate the reality of how AP was being diagnosed in the everyday clinical setting. Non-AP was defined as any patient diagnosed with CAP that was not documented as AP.

2.4. Data Collection

The following data were collected from medical records: patient demographics (age, sex), social history (whether they lived at home or in a care/nursing home), medical history (comorbidities, drugs, pneumonia within the past year, risk factors for multi-drug resistant organisms in pneumonia and healthcare-associated pneumonia (HCAP) [25,26]), presenting condition (CURB-65 score [27], pneumonia severity index [28], clinical frailty score [29], SARC-F score [30]), initial investigations undertaken in the emergency department (chest X-ray, chest computed tomography (CT), blood culture, sputum culture, urine pneumococcal and legionella antigen), initial diagnosis (AP or non-AP), other additional diagnoses, and management (initial antimicrobial treatment, initial NBM orders, speech and language therapist (SLT) referral, videofluoroscopic swallow study (VFSS), and fibreoptic endoscopic evaluation of swallowing (FEES)).

2.5. Antimicrobial Treatment

In the UK, each National Health Service (NHS) Trust has its own antimicrobial guidelines, depending on the drug sensitivity of the local microbiome. The guidelines are expected to be followed unless recommended otherwise. At the Lewisham and Greenwich NHS Trust (in which this study was performed), the recommended microbial treatment for pneumonia and lung infection is as follows:

1. CAP: amoxicillin, or amoxicillin and clarithromycin, depending on CURB-65 score (if allergic to penicillin: vancomycin and clarithromycin).
2. AP: amoxicillin, metronidazole, and gentamicin (if allergic to penicillin: teicoplanin, metronidazole, and gentamicin).
3. HAP (including CAP presenting within 1 month of discharge from hospital): amoxicillin and gentamycin, or amoxicillin and clavulanic acid, or amoxicillin, clavulanic acid, and amikacin (if allergic to penicillin: teicoplanin and gentamicin).
4. Infectious exacerbation of COPD: doxycycline.

Medical records were checked to see what antimicrobials were used, and whether the initial treatment consisted of the triple therapy for AP or not.

2.6. Statistical Analyses

Patients were separated into two groups according to the initial diagnosis: AP or non-AP. Patient background, symptoms, and management were compared between the two groups. Descriptive statistics for baseline data were presented as the percentage, median, and interquartile range. The Mann–Whitney U-test was used for continuous variables, and the chi-square test or Fisher's exact test for categorical variables. All data analyses were carried out using Microsoft Excel (2018, Microsoft Corporation, Redmond, WA, USA) and Social Science Statistics, 2022 [31,32]. A p value < 0.05 was considered to be statistically significant.

3. Results

3.1. Patient Selection

The patient selection process is shown in Figure 1. On the hospital database, a total of 1443 patients were listed as admitted with a primary or secondary diagnosis of pneumonia or pneumonitis during the study period. According to the exclusion criteria, 640 cases were excluded. This included 398 cases with COVID-19 pneumonitis, 137 with multiple admissions in the study period, 60 with no pneumonia according to medical records, 36 who had developed pneumonia after the admission, and 9 who were admitted for HAP. As a result, 803 cases were included in the study. Of the 803 cases, 134 (16.7%) were initially diagnosed as having aspiration pneumonia (AP group), and the remaining 669 cases constituted the non-AP group.

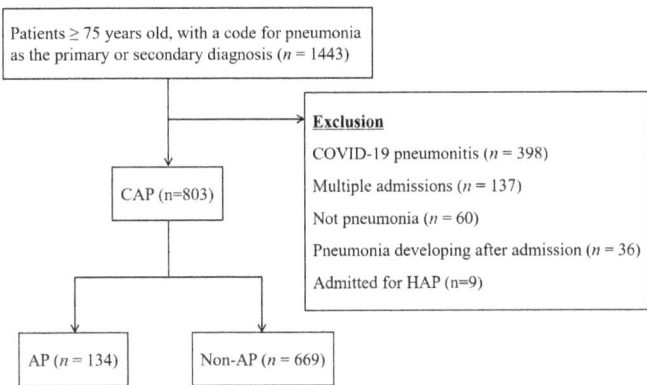

Figure 1. The patient selection process. A total of 1443 patients were listed as having a primary or secondary diagnosis of pneumonia or pneumonitis. According to the exclusion criteria, 640 cases were excluded. This included 398 cases with COVID-19 pneumonitis, 137 with multiple admissions in the study period, 60 with no pneumonia according to medical records, 36 who had developed pneumonia after the admission, and 9 who were admitted for hospital-acquired pneumonia (HAP). As a result, 803 cases of community-acquired pneumonia (CAP) were included in the study. Of the 803 cases, 134 were initially diagnosed as having aspiration pneumonia (AP group), and the remaining 669 cases constituted the non-AP group.

3.2. Patient Background

The patient demographic data are shown in Table 1. In total, there were 423 males (52.7%), and the median age was 84 years old (interquartile range: 80–89). There was no significant difference in the patient sex and age between the two groups. It was significantly more common for patients from the AP group to come from a care home or nursing home than in the non-AP group (29.9% vs. 11.3%, respectively, $p < 0.05$). Regarding their general well-being, the AP group had a significantly higher clinical frailty score (median 6 vs. 7) and SARC-F score (median 7 vs. 4) than in the non-AP group ($p < 0.05$). The patient demographic data excluding the 51 cases in which there was no detectable pneumonia on a CT scan (explained in 3.7) are shown in the Appendix A (Table A1). After exclusion, in the AP group, the comorbidities of ischemic/congestive cardiac conditions and type 2 diabetes mellitus were seen significantly more frequently in the AP group ($p < 0.05$), while having a history of pneumonia within 1 year of admission became non-significant ($p = 0.06$).

Table 1. Patient background and past medical history.

Factor	AP (n = 134)		Non-AP (n = 669)		p-Value
Background	n	%, IQR	n	%, IQR	
Male (n, %)	72	(53.7)	351	(52.5)	0.79
Age (median, IQR)	85	(80–90)	84	(80–89)	0.11
Care home/nursing home (n, %)	40	(29.9)	76	(11.4)	<0.001
Clinical frailty scale (median, IQR)	6	(5–7)	5	(4–6)	<0.001
SARC-F score (median, IQR)	7	(4–10)	4	(2–7)	<0.001
Past medical history, comorbidities					
Stroke (n, %)	28	(20.9)	102	(15.2)	0.11
Neurologic disorder (n, %)	23	(17.2)	28	(4.2)	<0.001
Dementia (n, %)	69	(51.5)	154	(23.0)	<0.001
Other mental disorder (n, %)	15	(11.2)	69	(10.3)	0.76
Gastroesophageal reflux disease (n, %)	8	(6.0)	28	(4.2)	0.36
Other gastroesophageal disorder (n, %)	17	(12.7)	53	(7.9)	0.07
Ischemic/congestive cardiac condition (n, %)	31	(23.1)	207	(30.9)	0.07
Type 2 diabetes mellitus (n, %)	22	(16.4)	161	(24.1)	0.05
Chronic respiratory disorder (n, %)	22	(16.4)	198	(29.6)	<0.05
Active cancer (n, %)	18	(13.4)	93	(13.9)	0.89
Head and neck cancer (n, %)	2	(1.5)	7	(1.0)	0.65
Immunodeficiency (n, %)	5	(3.7)	72	(10.8)	<0.05
Pneumonia within 1 year (n, %)	38	(28.4)	135	(20.2)	<0.05
Number of daily drugs (median, IQR)	6	(5–9)	7	(4–9)	0.13
Known dysphagia (n, %)	60	(44.8)	40	(6.0)	<0.001
Risk factors of multi-drug resistant pathogens					
Hospital admission ≥2 days in the past 90 days (n, %)	34	(25.4)	184	(27.5)	<0.001
Haemodialysis (n, %)	2	(1.5)	5	(0.7)	0.33
Intravenous antibiotic therapy in the last 90 days (n, %)	26	(19.4)	122	(18.2)	0.75

(AP: aspiration pneumonia, IQR: interquartile range).

3.3. Past Medical History

Data on past medical history are also shown in Table 1. Regarding comorbidities, those in the AP group were significantly more likely to have a history of neurologic conditions and dementia, and less likely to have a chronic respiratory disorder ($p < 0.05$). There was no significant difference between the two groups regarding the prevalence of stroke, other mental disorders (such as schizophrenia, depression, and epilepsy), gastroesophageal reflux disease (GORD), other gastroesophageal disorders, cardiac conditions, type 2 diabetes mellitus, active cancer, or head and neck cancer. As for risks of HCAP, the AP group had a significantly higher rate of having had pneumonia in the past year, a recent admission within 90 days ($p < 0.05$), and a significantly lower rate of immunodeficiency ($p < 0.05$) (haematologic condition, chemotherapy, or systemic steroids). There was no significant difference in the number of regular drugs, rate of haemodialysis, or having intravenous antibiotics/chemotherapy/wound care within 30 days. The AP group had a significantly higher rate of having known dysphagia (44.8% vs. 30.0%, $p < 0.05$).

3.4. Symptoms and Signs

Symptoms and signs at admission are shown in Table 2. There were significantly fewer patients in the AP group that complained of pleuritic pain, dyspnoea, and fever than in the non-AP group. There were significantly more patients in the AP group that had a history of symptoms suggestive of an aspiration: altered mental status, coughing on food, and vomiting. There were no significant differences in the two groups regarding cough or purulent sputum. No patient was assessed for their swallow before being diagnosed as AP or non-AP. With regard to the severity of pneumonia, the AP group had higher scores of CURB-65 and PSI than in the non-AP group ($p < 0.001$). The signs and symptoms of the patients, excluding the 51 cases in which there was no detectable pneumonia on a CT scan (explained in 3.7), are shown in the Appendix A (Table A2). There were no significant differences between the two tables.

Table 2. Presenting condition.

Factor	AP (n = 134)		Non-AP (n = 669)		p-Value
Symptoms	n	%, IQR	n	%, IQR	
Cough (n, %)	52	(38.8)	314	(46.9)	0.08
Purulent sputum (n, %)	30	(22.4)	166	(24.8)	0.55
Pleuritic pain (n, %)	1	(0.7)	33	(4.9)	<0.05
Dyspnoea (n, %)	40	(29.9)	380	(56.8)	<0.001
Fever (n, %)	27	(20.1)	191	(28.6)	<0.05
Coughing on oral intake (n, %)	32	(23.9)	12	(1.8)	<0.001
Vomiting (n, %)	60	(44.8)	43	(6.4)	<0.001
Altered mental status from baseline (n, %)	43	(32.1)	150	(22.4)	<0.05
Severity of the pneumonia					
CURB-65, median (n, IQR)	2	(2–3)	2	(1–2)	<0.001
Pneumonia severity index (median, IQR)	107	(95–128)	103	(84–119)	<0.001

(AP: aspiration pneumonia, IQR: interquartile range).

3.5. Diagnostic Investigations

The diagnostic investigations performed on admission regarding the pneumonia are shown in Table 3. In the AP group, blood culture, urine *Legionella* antigen tests, or chest CTs were significantly less likely to be performed than in the non-AP group. In both groups, sputum cultures and urine *S. pneumoniae* antigen tests were rarely performed, showing no significant difference in the frequency.

Table 3. Management following the diagnosis of pneumonia.

Factor	AP (n = 134)		Non-AP (n = 669)		p-Value
Further Investigations Performed	n	%	n	%	
Blood culture (n, %)	36	(26.9)	252	(37.7)	<0.05
Sputum culture (n, %)	6	(4.5)	40	(6.0)	0.49
Urine *S. pneumoniae* antigen (n, %)	0	(0)	11	(1.6)	0.23
Urine *Legionella* antigen (n, %)	2	(1.5)	46	(6.9)	<0.05
Chest CT scan (n, %)	12	(9.9)	118	(17.6)	<0.05
Antimicrobial treatment					
AP triple therapy (n, %)	71	(53.0)	19	(2.8)	<0.001
Actions on admission					
SLT referral (n, %)	94	(70.1)	119	(17.8)	<0.001
Nil by mouth orders (n, %)	70	(52.2)	49	(7.3)	<0.001
VFSS/FEES (n, %)	4	(3.0)	3	(0.4)	<0.05

(AP: aspiration pneumonia, IQR: interquartile range, CT: computed tomography. SLT: speech and language therapist, VFSS: videofluoroscopic swallow study, FEES: fibreoptic endoscopic evaluation of swallowing).

3.6. Alternative Diagnoses of CT

Among the 803 cases initially diagnosed with pneumonia, 130 underwent a CT scan upon the orders of the emergency physician or consultant in charge of admission. In most cases, the CTs were performed in order to rule out other diagnoses, such as pulmonary embolism or aortic dissection, or to investigate a suspected lung tumour. The scan was carried out within the following few days, and the results are shown in Table 4. In 51 of the 130 cases (39.2%), there was no pneumonia detected on the CT scans. In 56 cases

(43.1%), there was another diagnosis found on CT, such as a new cancer (13.1%), new lung metastases of a known cancer (6.2%), new lung nodules (2.3%), pleural effusion (4.6%), pulmonary oedema (2.3%), and others, such as interstitial lung disease and pneumothorax.

Table 4. Chest CT findings.

Findings	AP (n = 12)		Non-AP (n = 118)		Total (n = 130)	
	n	%	n	%	n	%
No pneumonia	4	(33.3)	47	(39.8)	51	(39.2)
Only pneumonia	6	(50.0)	56	(47.5)	62	(47.7)
Other diagnosis (+/− pneumonia)	5	(41.7)	51	(43.2)	56	(43.1)
Pulmonary embolism	0	(0)	14	(11.9)	14	(10.8)
Cancer, previously unidentified	1	(8.3)	16	(13.6)	17	(13.1)
Lung	1	(8.3)	12	(10.2)	13	(10.0)
Other (mediastinal, breast, liver, adrenal)	0	(0)	4	(3.4)	4	(3.1)
New lung metastasis of known cancer	2	(16.7)	6	(5.1)	8	(6.2)
New lung nodules (no pathological diagnosis)	0	(0)	3	(2.5)	3	(2.3)
Pleural effusion	0	(0)	6	(5.1)	6	(4.6)
Pulmonary oedema	0	(0)	3	(2.5)	3	(2.3)
Other (ILD, pneumothorax, emphysema, hiatal hernia)	2	(16.7)	3	(2.5)	5	(3.8)

(AP: aspiration pneumonia, ILD: interstitial lung disease).

3.7. Diagnosis of New Causative Conditions of Dysphagia and Aspiration

In a total of 35 cases (4.4%), a cause of dysphagia or aspiration not detected on admission was newly diagnosed later during the admission (Table 5). This constituted 13 cases (9.7%) from the AP group, and 22 cases (3.3%) from the non-AP group. The most commonly found were neurologic conditions (37.1%), including acute stroke and dementia. The second common cause was gastrointestinal conditions (28.6), including hiatal hernia and metastatic oesophageal obstruction. This was followed by drug-induced aspiration (17.1%), such as vomiting and altered mental status caused by hypercalcemia from osteoporosis treatment, or hypo-delirium due to antipsychotics or antidepressants. Other causes included head and neck conditions and cardiopulmonary conditions.

3.8. Management

The treatment and interventions are also shown in Table 3. Antimicrobial treatment was initiated in all patients except for one patient in the non-AP group who was recognised to be at the end of life and managed with palliative care. Antimicrobial regimens for AP were selected as the initial treatment significantly more often in the AP group than in the non-AP group (53.0% vs. 2.8%, respectively, $p < 0.05$).

In the AP group, NBM orders and speech and language therapist referrals were significantly more common than in the non-AP group ($p < 0.05$). VFSS/FEES were only performed in seven cases in total.

Table 5. Newly diagnosed causes of aspiration.

Causes	Total (n = 35)	
	n	(%)
Neurologic	13	(37.1)
Stroke	7	(20.0)
Dementia	5	(14.3)
Bell's palsy	1	(2.9)
Head and neck	3	(8.6)
Oral thrush	2	(5.7)
Laryngocele	1	(2.9)
Cardiopulmonary	3	(8.6)
First-degree atrioventricular block, syncope	1	(2.9)
Chronic obstructive lung disease	1	(2.9)
Obstructive sleep apnoea	1	(2.9)
Gastrointestinal	10	(28.6)
Hiatal hernia	4	(11.4)
Cholecystitis	1	(2.9)
Metastatic oesophageal obstruction	2	(5.7)
Oesophageal stenosis	1	(2.9)
Candida esophagitis	1	(2.9)
Achalasia	1	(2.9)
Drug induced	6	(17.1)
Hypercalcemia (osteoporosis treatment)	2	(5.7)
Hypo-delirium (antipsychotic, antidepressant)	2	(5.7)
Opioid toxicity	1	(2.9)
Nausea (iron supplement)	1	(2.9)

4. Discussion

We conducted a retrospective study to investigate factors utilised to differentiate AP from non-AP, and the consequential management of the two groups. Statistically significant differences were found between the groups, in factors leading to the diagnosis and their management, giving us an idea of how a diagnosis of AP is made and acted upon.

4.1. Diagnosis of Aspiration Pneumonia

Results showed that patients who were more likely to be diagnosed with AP than non-AP were those with the following factors: residing in care/ nursing homes, a history of neurologic conditions or dementia, previously diagnosed dysphagia, recent pneumonia, recent admission, frailer, and have a higher SARC-F score. As for symptoms, patients diagnosed with AP were significantly more likely to present with altered mental status, vomiting, or coughing on oral intake. No swallow function screenings or assessments were performed by the physicians diagnosing the pneumonia; no evaluation of airway clearance was taken into account. There were no cases in which diagnoses were postponed until after the SLT assessment. These findings suggest that clinicians may be more inclined to diagnose AP in a generally frail patient with more comorbidities who have symptoms suggestive of an aspiration than on the basis of a swallowing disorder. While these are common factors of AP, they are neither directly indicative of aspiration nor are they sufficient to make definitive diagnoses of AP. Assessments of the swallow and cough effectiveness are recommended [11]. Furthermore, vomiting imposes patients to aspiration pneumonitis, which is a chemical reaction of the lungs to the acidic aspirates of vomitus and differs from AP in diagnosis and management. In clinical practice, efforts to distinguish between the two may be neglected and antibiotics given, as it may seem to be the choice with less immediate risk.

On the contrary, patients with a coexisting chronic respiratory disorder were significantly less likely to be diagnosed as AP. These included COPD, interstitial lung disease, and bronchiectasis. When clinicians see patients with these coexisting respiratory conditions, they may tend to diagnose them with 'infective exacerbation of the underlying condition' and may be less likely to suspect aspiration as an additional underlying cause. However, it is known that chronic respiratory conditions [33], especially COPD [34], predispose patients to dysphagia. Moreover, aspiration can be the cause of infective exacerbations of COPD [35,36], exacerbations of interstitial lung disease [37,38], and adult bronchiectasis [39–41]. Therefore, a coexisting respiratory condition or an infective exacerbation should not discourage clinicians from suspecting aspiration; rather, it should prompt attention towards assessing the swallowing function and the possibility of the underlying aspiration.

4.2. Microbial Investigations

Following the diagnosis of AP or non-AP, further investigations were ordered by the emergency department, including blood and sputum cultures, and urine pneumococcal and legionella antigen tests. Blood cultures and urine legionella antigen tests were performed significantly less frequently in the AP group than the non-AP group. In any pneumonia, efforts to identify the causative organism and rule out other possible conditions are important for treatment. A diagnosis of AP or a state of frailty is not a reason against the microbial investigation. If anything, patients with AP, who often fall under the group of HCAP and are prone to resistant organisms [42], in addition to oral streptococcus species, require even more attention to identifying the causative organism. This is necessary, not only for the treatment of the presenting pneumonia but also for reference in the event of future infections and to prevent antimicrobial resistance or the nosocomial spread of infection.

Sputum culture was performed particularly infrequently in both groups. There may be a few reasons. In the UK, clinical practice is guided by the National Institute for Health and Care Excellence (NICE) guidelines [43], in addition to specific guidelines by each society. For CAP in adults treated in the hospital, the British Thoracic Society (BTS) guidelines state that 'sputum samples should be sent for culture and sensitivity tests from patients with CAP of moderate severity who are able to expectorate purulent samples and have not received prior antibiotic therapy' [16]. The NICE guidelines [43] and the *British Medical Journal* (BMJ) best practice guidelines [44] are also in line with this recommendation. It is suspected that a substantial proportion of these patients could not expectorate purulent samples initially or had received prior antibiotic therapy. Further, the COVID-19 pandemic has made it difficult to collect sputum in open environments such as emergency departments or normal wards. Nonetheless, sputum culture should be considered in the majority of cases of pneumonia, and this is a potential topic for quality improvement projects.

4.3. Further Investigations and Additional Diagnoses

Chest CTs were also performed significantly less in the AP group than in the non-AP group. CTs were ordered following the diagnosis of pneumonia, when a different pathophysiology was also suspected, such as a pulmonary embolism or a tumour. As a result of the scans, not only were a clinically substantial number of cases (39.2%) found to have no detectable pneumonia but also more than 40% were diagnosed with an alternative condition. Many were life-limiting, such as a newly identified cancer (13.1%), new metastases of what was thought to be stable cancer (6.2%), and pulmonary embolism (10.8%). In other cases, conditions that called for further investigations or interventions, such as pleural effusion, pulmonary oedema, and pneumothoraces were detected. This compares to the results of a previous study, in which 27.3% of patients admitted for CAP had a non-pneumonia diagnosis upon discharge [45]. Considering the high ratio of an alternative diagnosis being identified, there may be more undiagnosed cases in patients who did not undergo a CT scan, especially in the AP group, which was significantly less investigated. A diagnosis of AP or being frail does not justify fewer investigations. Patients diagnosed with AP who are generally frailer and have more comorbidities are also at risk of these conditions. Additionally, many patients with AP had been previously admitted for pneumonia, which also raises suspicion of a different condition, such as a tumour, empyema, or tuberculosis. In the clinical setting, once AP is suspected, it is unfortunately not uncommon for a clinician's mind to drift towards antibiotic treatment, NBM, and attaining a 'do not resuscitate' order, rather than logically rethinking their own clinical reasoning process and considering further investigation. If the history, physical examination, or other screening tests suggest the possibility of another condition, further investigation should be considered, including (but not limited to) CT scans.

4.4. Diagnosis of New Causes of Aspiration

Among the 803 cases, 35 cases (4.4%) were later diagnosed with a cause of aspiration during their hospital stay. These included life-threatening conditions, such as stroke or first-degree atrioventricular block, or treatable conditions, such as drug-induced aspirations. The non-AP group was less likely to be diagnosed with a cause of aspiration than the AP group (3.3% vs. 9.7%, respectively). This may, to some extent, be due to less investigation being performed to find a cause of aspiration in the non-AP group. If underlying causes of aspirations are left undiagnosed, it may lead to the progression of the condition, as well as recurrent pneumonia. It is difficult to accurately decide whether a patient has AP or non-AP with the limited information available at the initial patient contact. Therefore, when diagnosing older adults with pneumonia, it is essential to attain a detailed history of both acute and chronic symptoms with regard to possible aspiration, from the patient and family members or caregivers [46]. Rather than investigating the cause only in patients diagnosed with AP (of which the diagnosis may be inaccurate), it is recommended to consider the causes of aspiration in all pneumonia in older adults.

4.5. Management of the Patient

The choice of antimicrobial treatment differed between the two groups, understandably. The AP group was far more likely to be treated with the triple therapy antimicrobial regimen recommended for AP under the Trust guidelines. However, as few patients in the AP group underwent blood or sputum cultures, there is not enough information to confirm that this broad coverage was necessary. It may have put patients at risk of side effects, bacterial translocation, and future antimicrobial resistance. As the diagnosis of AP and non-AP remains ambiguous, deciding on antimicrobial treatment depending on these presumptive diagnoses entails clinical risk. Recently, it was recommended to start with narrow spectrum antimicrobials if the patient conditions allow and consider escalating the coverage if microbiology results are suggestive of resistant pathogens [17,44]. This is based on the increasing evidence suggesting a shift in causative pathogens of AP from anaerobic to aerobic organisms [47], and that anaerobic organisms causing AP are generally sensitive to narrow spectrum antimicrobials [15]. Therefore, it would be more clinically suitable if the initial antimicrobial treatment were to be selected by the patient's condition, background, and previous microbiology results whilst conducting new microbial investigations, rather than deciding the treatment on the basis of a presumptive diagnosis.

Patients with a diagnosis of AP were also more likely to be made NBM initially, which is also not an ideal method of management. Not only will depriving elderly patients of food put them at high risk of malnutrition and delirium, but the disuse of the swallowing function will only make their swallowing worse. Studies in older patients with AP have reported that putting patients on NBM is an independent predictive factor for prolonged treatment and a greater decline in swallowing function [48], while another study on older patients with pneumonia has reported that the lack of energy intake during the first week of admission was an independent risk factor for mortality, recovery, and recurrence [49]. Therefore, unless a patient is at a high risk of choking, distress, and hypoxia (such as the patient being unconscious or in severe respiratory distress), it is recommended to assess their swallowing function and continue some sort of oral intake. It is common practice for patients to be kept NBM over the weekend due to there being no SLTs to assess the swallowing function, or for fear of their condition worsening. However, there has been a report stating that starting oral intake on weekends showed a better prognosis on patients with AP diagnosis than starting on weekdays [50]. Initiating oral intake early and using other methods of nutrition therapy, such as nasogastric feeding, is important in the prevention of malnutrition and sarcopenia [51].

When aspiration is suspected, early SLT assessment and intervention has been known to improve patient outcomes [52]. SLTs were only referred in 17.8% of patients diagnosed with non-AP. However, as the diagnoses of non-AP were not based on any swallow assessments, it is suspected that there are many patients with underdiagnosed dysphagia and aspiration in this group. Studies show that in the older population, 27% of those in the community [53] and 55% of those hospitalized, up to 85.9% of those with dementia [54], and 91% hospitalized with CAP [55] have swallowing disorders. By presumptively diagnosing a patient with non-AP, we may be depriving them of the opportunity to identify and treat their dysphagia and prevent further pneumonia.

4.6. Suggestions of a Paradigm Shift in the Diagnosis of Pneumonia

Accurately diagnosing a patient is the first step towards treating them effectively and preventing any further conditions. By making a presumptive diagnosis of AP, clinicians are potentially denying patients appropriate investigation and management. We may be exposing them to inappropriate antibiotics and unwanted dietary restrictions, putting them at risk of unnecessary side effects and malnutrition. Moreover, by tentatively ruling out AP, we may be neglecting the opportunities to investigate the swallowing functions or underlying causes of aspiration in these patients.

AP is a highly commonly diagnosed condition in the elderly population, yet there is still no clear unified way to diagnose it. This conundrum, along with the results of our study, indicates that AP and non-AP are not straightforward black-or-white matters; rather, aspiration is an aetiology of pneumonia that can affect patients in different degrees. Therefore, when making a diagnosis of CAP, rather than concluding that a patient has AP or non-AP, it is more clinically relevant to explore to what extent aspiration contributes to pneumonia (Figure 2), along with other clinical aspects. We suggest this paradigm shift in the diagnosis of pneumonia in older persons. All patients with pneumonia should be considered for investigation according to the clinical appropriateness depending on their condition, rather than their 'label' of AP or non-AP. Clinicians should consider the clinical state of the patient, assess their ability to swallow and expectorate any aspiration, seek causative organisms, and investigate any underlying cause of dysphagia and aspiration or alternative diagnoses, as previously suggested [46]. To assess the extent of aspiration, simple individual screenings, such as the water swallow test or simple swallow provocation test, could be carried out, or mealtime assessments may be of use [56]. Depending on the screening results and availability, further bedside or instrumental assessment may be considered. There are also tools developed to guide the clinical management of pneumonia in older patients with a focus on AP, such as the Assessment of Swallowing Ability for Pneumonia (ASAP) [57] and the aspiration pneumonia cause investigation algorithm [58]. In pneumonia in older adults, rather than relying on a largely heterogeneous diagnostic term, the optimal care may be to manage patients according to attentive bedside examination and holistic assessment.

4.7. Strengths and Weaknesses of This Study

There are some limitations associated with this study. First, this was a single centre, retrospective study, performed in 2021, where the effects of the COVID-19 pandemic may still have some effect on the patient population. The situation may differ in other settings. However, this was a fairly large study involving an initial list of over 1400 patients with pneumonia, from a 521-bed acute hospital. To our knowledge, there have not been many studies undertaken on older adults diagnosed with AP in the UK, and this study is important to highlight current practices in the area. Second, diagnoses were extracted from medical records. Results may have been affected by how the diagnoses were made and documented. However, as the purpose of this study was to investigate what clinical factors appear to influence the diagnoses of AP and non-AP in the daily clinical setting, this was considered the feasible and optimal method for a retrospective study. We believe this is a meaningful step towards contemplating the challenging conundrum of diagnosing AP.

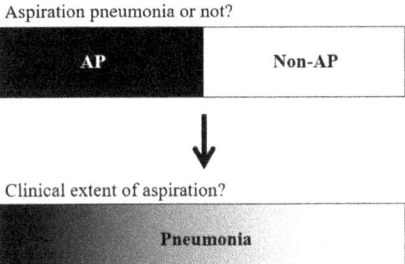

Figure 2. A paradigm shift in the diagnosis of pneumonia in older adults. Currently, the diagnosis of pneumonia in older adults is polarized among aspiration pneumonia (AP) or non-AP. We suggest the necessity of a paradigm shift in this process, where the diagnosis is pneumonia, and all older adults are assessed for the extent of clinical suspicion of aspiration.

5. Conclusions

In conclusion, older patients admitted for CAP were more likely to be diagnosed with AP if they were frailer and had more underlying conditions. The diagnosis of AP seemed to have led to the choice for broader antimicrobial coverage, NBM, and SLT referrals, rather than an assessment of the microbial risk factors or swallowing function. This study highlights the potential risks of a presumptive diagnosis and suggests a shift towards a more careful assessment of each patient's condition.

Author Contributions: Conceptualization, Y.Y. and D.G.S.; methodology, Y.Y. and D.G.S.; formal analysis, Y.Y.; investigation, Y.Y.; resources, Y.Y. and D.G.S.; data curation, Y.Y.; writing—original draft preparation, Y.Y.; writing—review and editing, D.G.S.; visualization, Y.Y.; supervision, D.G.S.; project administration, Y.Y.; funding acquisition, Y.Y. All authors have read and agreed to the published version of the manuscript.

Funding: The corresponding author is supported by the Japanese Respiratory Society Fellowship Grant of 2021. The authors received no other financial support for the research, authorship, and publication of this article. The authors declare that they have no competing interests.

Institutional Review Board Statement: Ethical approval was provided by the Lewisham and Greenwich NHS Trust as instituted by the Declaration of Helsinki.

Informed Consent Statement: Patient consent was waived due to the retrospective nature of this study.

Data Availability Statement: The data presented in this study are available upon request from the corresponding author. The data are not publicly available due to privacy and ethical reasons.

Acknowledgments: The authors would like to express their deepest gratitude to Ian Swaine at the University of Greenwich, and to the acute medical and elderly care team at Queen Elizabeth Hospital for their support.

Conflicts of Interest: The authors declare no conflict of interest. The funders had no role in the design of the study; in the collection, analyses, or interpretation of data; in the writing of the manuscript; or in the decision to publish the results.

Appendix A

Table A1. Patient background and past medical history, excluding patients without pneumonia, findings on CT.

Factor	AP (n = 130)		Non-AP (n = 622)		p-Value
Background	n	%, IQR	n	%, IQR	
Male (n, %)	70	(53.8)	326	(52.4)	0.76
Age (median, IQR)	85	(80–90)	84	(80–89)	0.11
Care home/nursing home (n, %)	40	(30.8)	72	(11.6)	<0.001
Clinical frailty scale (median, IQR)	6	(5–7)	5	(4–6)	<0.001
SARC-F score (median, IQR)	7	(4–10)	4	(2–7)	<0.001
Past medical history, comorbidities					
Stroke (n, %)	28	(21.5)	99	(15.9)	0.12
Neurologic disorder (n, %)	22	(16.9)	28	(4.5)	<0.001
Dementia (n, %)	68	(52.3)	147	(23.6)	<0.001
Other mental disorder (n, %)	15	(11.5)	63	(10.1)	0.63
Gastroesophageal reflux disease (n, %)	8	(6.2)	28	(4.5)	0.42
Other gastroesophageal disorder (n, %)	17	(13.1)	52	(8.4)	0.09
Ischemic/congestive cardiac condition (n, %)	29	(22.3)	198	(31.8)	<0.05
Type 2 diabetes mellitus (n, %)	21	(16.2)	152	(24.4)	<0.05
Chronic respiratory disorder (n, %)	21	(16.2)	184	(29.6)	<0.05
Active cancer (n, %)	17	(13.1)	85	(13.7)	0.86
Head and neck cancer (n, %)	2	(1.5)	6	(1.0)	0.63
Immunodeficiency (n, %)	5	(3.8)	66	(10.6)	<0.05
Pneumonia within 1 year (n, %)	36	(27.7)	126	(20.3)	0.06
Number of daily drugs (median, IQR)	6	(5–9)	7	(4–9)	0.07
Known dysphagia (n, %)	60	(46.2)	40	(6.4)	<0.001
Risk factors of multi-drug resistant pathogens					
Hospital admission ≥2 days in the past 90 days (n, %)	33	(25.4)	173	(27.8)	<0.001
Haemodialysis (n, %)	2	(1.5)	5	(0.8)	0.35
Intravenous antibiotic therapy in the last 90 days (n, %)	25	(19.2)	113	(18.2)	0.78

(AP: aspiration pneumonia, IQR: interquartile range).

Table A2. Presenting condition, excluding patients without pneumonia findings on CT.

Factor	AP (n = 130)		Non-AP (n = 622)		p-Value
Symptoms	n	%, IQR	n	%, IQR	
Cough (n, %)	51	(39.2)	293	(47.1)	0.08
Purulent sputum (n, %)	30	(23.1)	151	(24.3)	0.55
Pleuritic pain (n, %)	1	(0.8)	28	(4.5)	<0.05
Dyspnoea (n, %)	40	(30.8)	350	(56.3)	<0.001
Fever (n, %)	26	(20.0)	181	(29.1)	<0.05
Coughing on oral intake (n, %)	31	(23.8)	12	(1.9)	<0.001
Vomiting (n, %)	57	(43.8)	42	(6.8)	<0.001
Altered mental status from baseline (n, %)	43	(33.1)	144	(23.2)	<0.05
Severity of the pneumonia					
CURB-65, median (n, IQR)	2	(2–3)	2	(1–2)	<0.001
Pneumonia severity index (median, IQR)	107	(95–128)	103	(85–119)	<0.05

(AP: aspiration pneumonia, IQR: interquartile range).

References

1. Marin, S.; Serra-Prat, M.; Ortega, O.; Clavé, P. Healthcare-related cost of oropharyngeal dysphagia and its complications pneumonia and malnutrition after stroke: A systematic review. *BMJ Open* **2020**, *10*, e031629. [CrossRef] [PubMed]
2. Sun, X.; Douiri, A.; Gulliford, M. Pneumonia incidence trends in UK primary care from 2002 to 2017: Population-based cohort study. *Epidemiol. Infect.* **2019**, *147*, e263. [CrossRef] [PubMed]
3. Marik, P.E. Aspiration Pneumonitis and Aspiration Pneumonia. *N. Engl. J. Med.* **2001**, *344*, 665–671. [CrossRef] [PubMed]
4. Feldman, C.; Anderson, R. Epidemiology, virulence and management of pneumococcus. *F1000Research* **2016**, *5*, 2320. [CrossRef] [PubMed]
5. Manabe, T.; Teramoto, S.; Tamiya, N.; Okochi, J.; Hizawa, N. Risk Factors for Aspiration Pneumonia in Older Adults. *PLoS ONE* **2015**, *10*, e0140060. [CrossRef]
6. Pneumonia Statistics. Available online: https:statistics:blf.org.uk/pneumonia (accessed on 21 July 2022).
7. Teramoto, S.; Fukuchi, Y.; Sasaki, H.; Sato, K.; Sekizawa, K.; Matsuse, T.; Japanese Study Group on Aspiration Pulmonary Disease. High incidence of aspiration pneumonia in community- and hospital-acquired pneumonia in hospitalized patients: A multicenter, prospective study in Japan. *J. Am. Geriatr. Soc.* **2008**, *56*, 577–579. [CrossRef]
8. Ortega, O.; Martín, A.; Clavé, P. Diagnosis and Management of Oropharyngeal Dysphagia Among Older Persons, State of the Art. *J. Am. Med. Dir. Assoc.* **2017**, *18*, 576–582. [CrossRef]
9. Langmore, S.; Terpenning, M.S.; Schork, A.; Chen, Y.; Murray, J.T.; Lopatin, D.E.; Loesche, W.J. Predictors of Aspiration Pneumonia: How Important Is Dysphagia? *Dysphagia* **1998**, *13*, 69–81. [CrossRef]
10. Yamaya, M.; Yanai, M.; Ohrui, T.; Arai, H.; Sasaki, H. Interventions to Prevent Pneumonia Among Older Adults. *J. Am. Geriatr. Soc.* **2001**, *49*, 85–90. [CrossRef]
11. Okazaki, T.; Suzukamo, Y.; Miyatake, M.; Komatsu, R.; Yaekashiwa, M.; Nihei, M.; Izumi, S.; Ebihara, T. Respiratory Muscle Weakness as a Risk Factor for Pneumonia in Older People. *Gerontology* **2021**, *67*, 581–590. [CrossRef]
12. Okazaki, T.; Ebihara, S.; Mori, T.; Izumi, S.; Ebihara, T. Association between sarcopenia and pneumonia in older people. *Geriatr. Gerontol. Int.* **2019**, *20*, 7–13. [CrossRef] [PubMed]
13. Hayashi, M.; Iwasaki, T.; Yamazaki, Y.; Takayasu, H.; Tateno, H.; Tazawa, S.; Kato, E.; Wakabayashi, A.; Yamaguchi, F.; Tsuchiya, Y.; et al. Clinical features and outcomes of aspiration pneumonia compared with non-aspiration pneumonia: A retrospective cohort study. *J. Infect. Chemother.* **2014**, *20*, 436–442. [CrossRef] [PubMed]
14. Yoon, H.-Y.; Shim, S.S.; Kim, S.J.; Lee, J.H.; Chang, J.H.; Lee, S.H.; Ryu, Y.J. Long-Term Mortality and Prognostic Factors in Aspiration Pneumonia. *J. Am. Med. Dir. Assoc.* **2019**, *20*, 1098–1104.e4. [CrossRef] [PubMed]
15. Metlay, J.P.; Waterer, G.W.; Long, A.C.; Anzueto, A.; Brozek, J.; Crothers, K.; Cooley, L.A.; Dean, N.C.; Fine, M.J.; Flanders, S.A.; et al. Diagnosis and treatment of adults with community-acquired pneumonia. An official clinical practice guideline of the american thoracic society and infectious diseases society of America. *Am. J. Respir. Crit. Care Med.* **2019**, *200*, e45–e67. [CrossRef]
16. Lim, W.S.; Baudouin, S.V.; George, R.C.; Hill, A.T.; Jamieson, C.; Le Jeune, I.; Macfarlane, J.T.; Read, R.C.; Roberts, H.J.; Levy, M.L.; et al. BTS guidelines for the management of community acquired pneumonia in adults: Update 2009. *Thorax* **2009**, *64*, iii1–iii55. [CrossRef]
17. The Japanese Respiratory Society. *The JRS Guidelines for the Management of Pneumonia in Adults*; Medical Review Co.: Tokyo, Japan, 2017. (In Japanese)
18. Marrie, T.J.; Durant, H.; Yates, L. Community-Acquired Pneumonia Requiring Hospitalization: 5-Year Prospective Study. *Clin. Infect. Dis.* **1989**, *11*, 586–599. [CrossRef]
19. Komiya, K.; Ishii, H.; Kadota, J.-I. Healthcare-associated Pneumonia and Aspiration Pneumonia. *Aging Dis.* **2015**, *6*, 27–37. [CrossRef] [PubMed]
20. Wei, C.; Cheng, Z.; Zhang, L.; Yang, J. Microbiology and prognostic factors of hospital- and community-acquired aspiration pneumonia in respiratory intensive care unit. *Am. J. Infect. Control* **2013**, *41*, 880–884. [CrossRef] [PubMed]
21. Almirall, J.; Boixeda, R.; de la Torre, M.C.; Torres, A. Aspiration pneumonia: A renewed perspective and practical approach. *Respir. Med.* **2021**, *185*, 106485. [CrossRef]
22. Komiya, K.; Rubin, B.K.; Kadota, J.-I.; Mukae, H.; Akaba, T.; Moro, H.; Aoki, N.; Tsukada, H.; Noguchi, S.; Shime, N.; et al. Prognostic implications of aspiration pneumonia in patients with community acquired pneumonia: A systematic review with meta-analysis. *Sci. Rep.* **2016**, *6*, 38097. [CrossRef]
23. Yoshimatsu, Y.; Melgaard, D.; Westergren, A.; Skrubbeltrang, C.; Smithard, D.G. The Diagnosis of Aspiration Pneumonia: A Systematic Review. *Eur. Geriatr. Med.* **2022**; *in press*.
24. Kalil, A.C.; Metersky, M.L.; Klompas, M.; John Muscedere, J.; Sweeney, D.A.; Palmer, L.B.; Napolitano, L.M.; O'Grady, N.P.; Bartlett, J.G.; Carratalà, J.; et al. Management of Adults with Hospital-acquired and Ventilator-associated Pneumonia: 2016 Clinical Practice Guidelines by the Infectious Diseases Society of America and the American Thoracic Society. *Clin. Infect. Dis.* **2016**, *63*, e61–e111. [CrossRef] [PubMed]
25. Gidal, A.; Barnett, S. Risk Factors Associated with Multidrug-Resistant Pneumonia in Nonhospitalized Patients. *Fed. Pr. Healthc.* **2018**, *35*, 16–18.
26. Shindo, Y.; Ito, R.; Kobayashi, D.; Ando, M.; Ichikawa, M.; Shiraki, A.; Goto, Y.; Fukui, Y.; Iwaki, M.; Okumura, J.; et al. Risk Factors for Drug-Resistant Pathogens in Community-acquired and Healthcare-associated Pneumonia. *Am. J. Respir. Crit. Care Med.* **2013**, *188*, 985–995. [CrossRef]

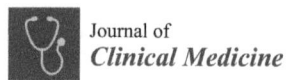

Review

Comprehensive Approaches to Aspiration Pneumonia and Dysphagia in the Elderly on the Disease Time-Axis

Takae Ebihara

Department of Geriatric Medicine, Graduate School of Medicine, Kyorin University, Tokyo 181-8611, Japan; takae-ebi@ks.kyorin-u.ac.jp; Tel.: +81-422-47-5511; Fax: +81-422-44-0849

Abstract: Pneumonia in the elderly has been increasing on an annual basis. To a greater or lesser extent, aspiration is a major contributor to the development of pneumonia in the elderly. Antimicrobials alone are not sufficient for the treatment of pneumonia, and the condition may become intractable or even recur repeatedly. In addition, some patients with pneumonia may have no problems with eating, while others are unable to receive the necessary nutrition due to severe dysphagia. It has recently been found that pneumonia decreases both the muscle mass and strength of the swallowing and respiratory muscles, a condition named pneumonia-associated sarcopenia. This contributes to a pathophysiological time-axis of aspiration pneumonia and dysphagia in the elderly, in which silent aspiration leads to the development of pneumonia, and further to dysphagia, malnutrition, and low immunity. Therefore, it is recommended that the treatment and prevention of developing pneumonia should also differ according to an individual's placement in the disease time-axis. In particular, approaches for preventing aspiration based on scientific findings are able to be implemented at home.

Keywords: aspiration pneumonia; pneumonia-related sarcopenia; TRP agonist; nutrition; time-axis

1. Introduction

As Sir Osler stated, "Pneumonia is an old man's friend". Pneumonia among the elderly has been increasing in advanced countries, where populations are ageing at an accelerating rate. As most deaths from pneumonia in the elderly are attributed to aspiration pneumonia (AsP), its diagnosis, treatment, and prevention are important clinical topics. Clinically, AsP can be divided into 'overt aspiration', in which the aspiration is evident, and 'silent aspiration', in which the aspiration is not apparent. Videofluoroscopy is capable of detecting both overt and silent aspiration, but is unable to detect "micro-aspiration"; that is, the aspiration of small amounts of oropharyngeal secretions due to a depressed swallowing reflex during sleep. Micro-aspiration may or may not present with symptoms suggestive of aspiration, such as coughing. In particular, micro-aspiration without symptoms (i.e., silent aspiration) is important in the development of pneumonia. On the other hand, choking during a meal due to aspirated food debris or its detection in the sputum (macro-aspiration) is considered overt aspiration. As elderly patients with pneumonia often present with non-specific symptoms, such as general malaise, impaired consciousness, and loss of appetite, the onset of pneumonia may only be detected after a chest X-ray; moreover, the disease is often severe [1]. Therefore, it is important to determine the presence or absence of silent aspiration and the means for its prevention for the treatment of pneumonia in the elderly.

2. Prevalence

Pneumonia is a disease with high mortality and morbidity worldwide. In Japan, pneumonia is the leading cause of death in people aged 65 years and over, and is particularly prominent in men aged 80 years and over [2].

Despite AsP generally being more likely to occur in the elderly, the prevalence of AsP may be under-estimated. The prevalence of AsP in the USA has been estimated to be 5–15%

among hospitalized patients with community- and hospital-acquired pneumonia [3,4]. Meanwhile, in a cross-sectional national survey of Japan, the prevalence rates of AsP in hospitalized community- and hospital-acquired pneumonia were 60.1% and 86.7%, respectively; this further increased with age, accounting for about 85% in those aged 80–89 years and more than 90% in those aged 90 years and older [5]. This Japanese survey involved a swallowing function test, in order to detect not only overt aspiration but also silent aspiration, and it was found that aspiration is greatly associated with the cause of pneumonia in the elderly. From this study report, it may be no exaggeration to say that most pneumonia in the elderly is AsP.

3. Mechanism

The main responsible factor in the development of AsP is the deterioration of the swallowing reflex and cough reflex sensitivity due to reduced release of the neurotransmitter substance P from the nerve endings of the glossopharyngeal and the vagal nerves [6] (Figure 1).

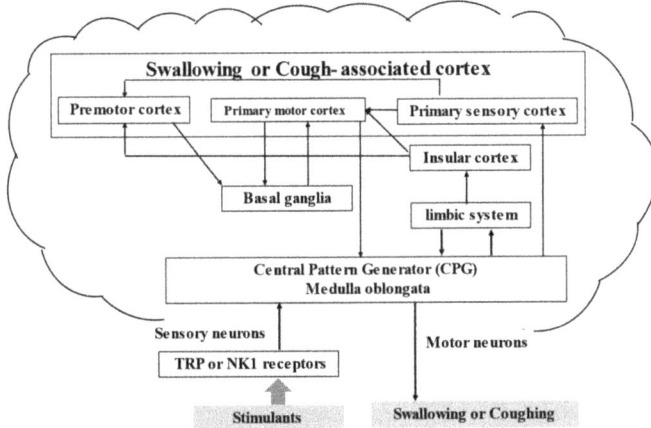

Figure 1. Swallowing, coughing, and the brain. Abbreviations: TRP, transient receptor potential; NK1, neurokinin 1.

3.1. Cough Reflex Sensitivity

Coughs are provoked by the ligand substance P of the neurokinin 1 receptor, located in the respiratory tract and in the nucleus tractus solitarii of the brainstem [7–9]. In support, selective neurokinin 1 antagonists have been found to completely suppress coughing in a study in guinea pigs [10,11]. Another animal study has shown that aerosols of a substance P antagonist inhibited acetylcholine- and histamine-induced coughs, which are bronchoconstricting agents [12]. Additionally, coughing was induced through the inhalation of substance P by patients with pulmonary fibrosis [13].

However, contrary to general expectations, geriatric wards—where pneumonia patients are mainly hospitalized—are often quiet, with few coughing patients. The cough reflex sensitivity induced by chemical stimulants is typically blunted in elderly patients with repeated pneumonia [14]. Specifically, the threshold for coughing to citric acid mist in elderly people with repeated pneumonia was a concentration greater than 1.35 log mg mL^{-1}, compared to less than 0.5 log mg mL^{-1} in non-pneumonia patients [15].

3.2. Swallowing Reflex

Similar to the blunted cough reflex sensitivity, the triggering of the swallowing reflex is also blunted in elderly patients with repeated pneumonia; in particular, the latency of the swallowing reflex in patients with repeated pneumonia has been found to be >5 s [15].

The provocation of the swallowing reflex was mediated by substance P in a capsaicin concentration-dependent manner [16].

3.3. Lacunar Infarction and the Upper Respiratory Protective Reflexes

The blunted swallowing reflex and cough reflex sensitivity have been associated with lacunar infarction in the basal ganglia [17]. In patients with bilateral lacunar infarction, the swallowing reflex latency is significantly higher than in other patients with unilateral or no lacunar infarction, and the swallowing reflex latency gradually increases, not only during the day but also at night, with a greater rate of change from daytime than in other patients. Additionally, the incidence of aspiration—assessed using indium chloride—was reported to be higher in elderly patients with bilateral lacunar infarction [18]. The cough reflex sensitivity in the elderly with lacunar infractions has also been shown to be depressed. Furthermore, both the swallowing and coughing reflexes, among others, were greatly impaired in those who developed AsP [17].

The production of substance P is associated with dopamine metabolism. In animal models pre-treated with dopamine 1 receptor antagonists, the provocation of the swallowing reflex was delayed, and the swallowing frequency was increased with exogenously administered substance P, while substance P antagonists decreased the swallowing frequency. In other words, the swallowing reflex and swallowing frequency are substance P-dependent, while substance P is dopamine-dependent [19]. Taken together, the presence of lacunar infarcts may suggest that the blunted swallowing reflex latency and cough reflex sensitivity are due to the reduced release of substance P.

3.4. Brain and Swallowing

Reduced activity in the insular cortex has been reported in elderly patients with repeated AsP [20]. Functional cerebral imaging during swallowing in healthy adults has shown that the primary motor and sensory areas are most activated, with additional bilateral activation of the anterior cingulate cortex, insula and basal ganglia capsules, and globus pallidus and substantia nigra [21–23]. Therefore, the bilateral inactivation of the insula and basal ganglia may contribute to the development of AsP.

3.5. Breathing and Swallowing

Sensory inputs to the sensory nerves reach the medulla oblongata afferentially and integrate the activity of swallowing-related muscles through central pattern generators (CPGs), such that breathing and swallowing can be appropriately coordinated. Natural swallowing begins with laryngeal closure after inspiration (post-inspiratory activity). In more detail, glutamatergic–cholinergic neurons and excitatory networks that generate neural correlates of post-inspiratory activity and inhibitory neural networks, through gamma-aminobutyric acid, contribute to the regulation of timing involved in inspiration [24]. Furthermore, inputs to the CPG from the cortical swallowing area (including the insular cortex) have also been reported to modulate these coordinated respiratory–swallowing movements. In other words, failure to provoke the upper respiratory protective reflex may interfere with the inspiratory and post-inspiratory coordination, which may contribute to the onset of AsP [25].

3.6. Comorbidities Modifying the Development of Pneumonia

Several comorbidities contribute to the development of AsP. Gastrointestinal diseases with organic problems and dysfunction are representative comorbidities of AsP. In addition to age-related gastro-oesophageal motility disorders, post-operative status following gastrectomy leads to a predisposition to aspiration of gastrointestinal contents due to reflux [26]. Furthermore, gastric reflux is more likely to occur in elderly people with hiatal hernia of the oesophagus, which has been estimated to affect one in two women over 80 years of age; furthermore, acidity (especially below pH 4) increases the swallowing reflex latency in a negatively pH-dependent manner [27]. The relationship between gastric acid and the swallowing reflex is considered as a factor affecting the occurrence of AsP in this paper. Elderly people often present with chronic constipation, some of whom may vomit due to impaired bowel peristalsis, leading to chemical pneumonitis [28]. Other factors contributing to the development of AsP have been previously reported, including dementia, physical activity impairment, gender, smoking history, decreased oral intake, and drugs such as neuroleptics, which exacerbate the swallowing reflex by lowering serum substance P, resulting in the development of AsP [29,30].

Anticholinergics are also a risk factor for AsP, as the incidence of AsP has been reported to increase in proportion to the intensity of anticholinergic side-effects such as falls, xerostomia, dry eyes, dizziness, confusion, and constipation [31]. It has also been reported that acid suppressants, such as histamine 2 inhibitors and proton pump inhibitors, tend to increase the pH of gastric juice, thereby altering the gastric flora and even the mesopharyngeal microbiota, facilitating the development of AsP [32,33]. Taken together, drugs with antidopaminergic, bowel peristalsis-reducing, or anticholinergic effects, as well as other drugs that alter the gastric microbiota, should be withdrawn and replaced by drugs with other mechanisms of action.

3.7. Pneumonia-Associated Sarcopenia

Initially, sarcopenia is defined as an age-related decrease in skeletal muscle mass and strength [34]. As a muscle atrophy other than ageing, it is already well-known in mouse models that hypoxia (8 h/day, 30 cycles/hour, FiO_2 nadir = 6%) reduces the contractile properties of the diaphragm, especially as a result of muscle atrophy due to increased autophagy, prompting a compensatory metabolic adaptation that increases fatigue tolerance [35].

Since sarcopenia (assessed by grip strength and lower leg circumference) was reported as a risk factor for the development of community-acquired pneumonia in the elderly [36], a number of reports have revealed the association between pneumonia and sarcopenia.

Acute inflammation and chronic inflammation of the lungs are known to cause muscle atrophy [37]. In a retrospective database study of 739 ventilated patients, a reduction in muscle mass was observed, of which about half also had reduced muscle fiber density [38]. Furthermore, it has recently been shown that chronic aspiration and pneumonia cause a reduction in the cross-sectional area of the muscle fibers, including swallowing and respiratory muscles. In an animal model of lipopolysaccharide-induced aspiration, it has been shown that muscle atrophy of the tongue is induced by autophagy, thinning of the diaphragm by inflammatory cytokine production and the ubiquitin–proteasome pathway, and atrophy of the anterior tibialis muscle—which represents skeletal muscle—by both pathways [39].

In elderly patients hospitalized with AsP, the cross-sectional area of the erector spinae muscle, a respiratory accessory muscle, has been reported to decrease by approximately 80% during the time between admission and pneumonia healing. Further, our previous cross-sectional prospective cohort study has shown that both the inspiratory and expiratory respiratory muscle strength and trunk muscle mass were lower in the elderly with pneumonia compared to those with other respiratory diseases, which can, thus, be considered as risk factors for the development and recurrence of pneumonia [40]. With regard to swallowing, it has also been reported that the swallowing and chewing ability is related to the whole-body muscle mass; that poor swallowing ability, as assessed by the water-swallowing test, is mildly related to the upper arm circumference; and that the tongue muscle mass and tongue pressure are significantly lower in people with dysphagia than those without [41–45].

Finally, chronic aspiration and pneumonia lead to decreases in muscle mass and strength, resulting in reduced swallowing capacity, dysphagia due to a reduced expiratory cough peak flow, respiratory muscle fatigue, and reduced respiratory ventilation efficiency. Pneumonia-related sarcopenia leads to a negative pattern of refractory and recurrent pneumonia, as well as further progression of sarcopenia.

3.8. End-of-Life in Aspiration Pneumonia and Dysphagia

To date, no studies have examined impaired upper respiratory protective reflexes (e.g., the swallowing reflex and cough reflex sensitivity) as a risk factor for mortality in the elderly. We have recently reported that under-nutrition and an impaired swallowing reflex and cough reflex sensitivity—but not an impaired oral intake capacity—were predictors of death within 90 days in elderly AsP patients [46]. Furthermore, cholecystitis and cholangitis frequently occur in the terminal stages of the disease, which are thought to be due to the loss of gallbladder contractility caused by reduced lipid intake due to fasting, which increases the viscosity of the bile, causing it to become sludgy and unable to be expelled [47].

3.9. Pathophysiological Time-Axis of Aspiration Pneumonia and Dysphagia

A noteworthy emerging finding is the time-course of AsP and dysphagia in the elderly: starting with a delayed swallowing reflex, the sensitivity of the cough reflex gradually blunts and AsP develops. The onset of AsP leads to muscle atrophy and weakness of the swallowing and respiratory muscles; that is, a state of pneumonia-associated sarcopenia. Decreases in upper airway protective reflexes and sarcopenia are likely to lead to recurrent pneumonia and further sarcopenia progression, resulting in feeding difficulties and under-nutrition. The inability to meet nutritional requirements, whether by oral intake or other nutritional routes, can be considered terminal (Figure 2).

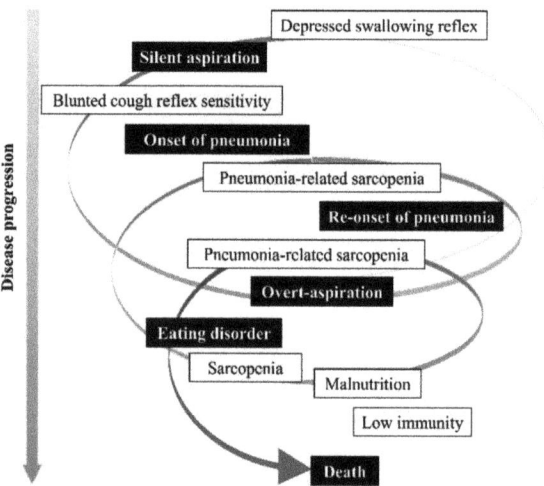

Figure 2. Time-axis of aspiration pneumonia and dysphagia in the elderly.

4. Comprehensive Preventive Approach

In addition to adequate antibiotic treatment, comprehensive prophylaxis is important in the treatment of AsP. Specifically, key points include the administration of drugs that promote the production and release of substance P or inhibit its degradation, the improvement of the gastrointestinal motility, the withdrawal of drugs that increase the risk of developing AsP, and nursing and care based on scientific knowledge.

4.1. Pharmacological Preventive Approach

4.1.1. Angiotensin-Converting Enzyme Inhibitors

Dry cough is an adverse symptom of angiotensin-converting enzyme inhibitors (ACE-I) [48]. It is well-known that bradykinin and substance P are the causative agents of coughing, and this side-effect is more common in peri- and post-menopausal women [11,48]. In a study of menopausal animal models, ACE-I increased the cough reflex sensitivity, while the coughs were significantly diminished by substance P antagonists [11]. Human studies have reported higher cough reflex sensitivity and substance P concentrations in the sputum in those taking ACE-I compared to non-users [49]. The swallowing reflex in humans was also significantly improved within two weeks after ACE-I medication [50]. In a three-year prospective cohort study of elderly patients with cerebrovascular disease, conducted on the basis of the results of this study, the incidence of pneumonia in the ACE-I treated group was significantly reduced compared with the control, Ca channel blocker, and diuretic groups, suggesting that ACE-I is effective for the prevention of pneumonia [51,52]. Taken together, in clinical situations, ACE-I may be a suitable antihypertensive for hypertensive patients with a history of aspiration or AsP.

4.1.2. Dopamine-Release-Stimulating Agent

As discussed above, dysfunction of the dopaminergic neurons results in a deteriorated swallowing reflex [19], which may lead to the development of pneumonia [17,18]. Amantadine acts as an antagonist at N-methyl-D-aspartate-type glutamate receptors, increasing dopamine release and inhibiting its re-uptake.

In a three-year prospective cohort study, elderly patients with lacunar infarction who were taking amantadine orally had a significantly lower incidence of pneumonia than those not taking the drug, suggesting that dopamine enhancement is effective against the development of pneumonia [53].

4.1.3. Combination of Dopamine-Release-Stimulating Agent and ACE Inhibitor

The treatment of pneumonia with ACE-I or amantadine, as well as antimicrobials, significantly decreased the number of antimicrobial treatment days, hospitalization days, healthcare costs, incidence of methicillin-resistant staphylococcus aureus, and hospital mortality over a one-year period [54]. In another case report, a patient with advanced Alzheimer's disease was treated with amantadine, levodopa, and ACE-I, and went from being lethargic and anorexic to smiling and talking to their carers, with increased appetite and improved eating disorders, resulting in a recovery of body mass index to the normal range [55]. Therefore, the addition of ACE-I and dopamine-releasing agents may be effective for the prevention of pneumonia in elderly patients with recurrent pneumonia and eating disorders.

4.1.4. Phosphodiesterase-III Inhibitors

It has been reported that a one-year intervention in a cilostazol-treated group (an anti-platelet drug with a phosphodiesterase-III-inhibitory effect) led to an approximately twice as low incidence of pneumonia compared to the non-treated group [56]. Cilostazol not only prevents a high rate of recurrent stroke, but also increases the cerebral blood flow in swallowing-related cerebral regions. It has been reported that cilostazol prevented the incidence of stroke-related pneumonia in patients with acute ischaemic stroke upon tube feeding compared to those without [57,58].

4.1.5. 5-Hydroxytryptamine$_4$ Receptor Agonist

A one-year prospective cohort study of post-gastrectomy elderly patients with cerebrovascular disease showed a lower incidence of pneumonia in mosapride-treated patients compared with non-treated patients [59]. Mosapride stimulates 5-hydroxytryptamin$_4$ receptors in the gastrointestinal tract's intrinsic plexus and promotes gastrointestinal motility. In patients receiving gastrostomy feeding, mosapride administration has been shown to be a significant preventive factor for pneumonia [60]. On the other hand, intestinal motility enhancers containing mosapride, unlike cilostazol, did not show a preventive effect on the development of stroke-related pneumonia. In other words, mosapride may prevent the development of pneumonia related specifically to gastrointestinal dysmotility.

4.2. Non-Pharmacological Approach: How to Prevent Aspiration at Home

4.2.1. Physical Properties of the Meal

Viscoelasticity, cohesion, and hardness are the three pillars of a texture-modified diet for dysphagia. In clinical settings, foods are typically blended or chopped and served in various thickened liquids (e.g., nectar-, honey-, or paste-thickened), or in the form of a mousse, pudding, or jelly. It has been reported that thickened liquids have significantly faster oral transit times than water but slower pharyngeal transit times, and may leave significant residue [61]. Therefore, can thickening really reduce the incidence of pneumonia? A three-month prospective cohort study has reported that nectar- and honey-thickened liquids decreased aspiration but not the incidence of pneumonia or death, while honey-thickened liquids increased dehydration and anorexia [62]. This means that thickening should not be over-estimated, as texture-modified diets for older people with dysphagia are effective in preventing aspiration, but do not reduce the incidence of pneumonia or death.

4.2.2. Stimulation of Transient Receptor Potential (TRP) Receptor

The temperature of and spices in meals are also important in preventing aspiration.

4.2.2.1. Temperature of the Meal

The temperature of the meal is an important factor. Temperature-sensitive transient receptor potential (TRP) channels exist in the neural endings of the glossopharyngeal and the vagal sensory branch; TRPV1 receptors respond to hot temperatures (above 60 °C) and TRPM8 receptors to cold temperatures (below 17 °C). Both hot and cold temperatures dramatically sharpen the swallowing reflex, which is delayed by more than 10 s to within the normal range. It is, therefore, advisable to serve food at distinct temperatures, such as hot or cold [63]. For patients with dysphagia, meals served at room temperature are more likely to induce aspiration.

4.2.2.2. Spices

Capsaicin, the pungent component of chilli peppers, is a TRPV1 agonist that triggers the cough or swallow reflex by releasing SP from sensory nerve endings, especially when applied at concentrations of 10^{-9} to 10^{-11} log M/mL, which can improve the swallowing reflex latency in a concentration-dependent manner [16]. Similarly, menthol, a cooling component of mint and a TRPM8 agonist, can also improve the swallowing reflex latency in a concentration-dependent manner at concentrations from 10^{-2} M to 10^{-4} M, especially at concentrations higher than 10^{-3} M, with a significantly shorter reflex than ice water [64].

4.2.3. Aromatherapy

Older people with repeated AsP often show reduced activities of the bilateral insular cortex [20]. Increasing the insular cortical activity, therefore, may serve as a preventive measure against AsP. Piperine, a component of black pepper, is also a TRPV1 agonist that shortens the swallowing reflex, while odour components extracted from the peel activate the insular cortex via the olfactory cortex. In a one-month randomized controlled trial of institutionalized elderly residents, olfactory stimulation with black pepper aroma for one minute before each meal significantly improved the swallowing reflex and the number of swallowing movements, as well as blood flow in the insular cortex upon cerebral single-photon emission computed tomography [65]. The smell-based prevention of aspiration is easy to introduce not only to patients with chronic aspiration or repeated pneumonia, but also to patients with impaired consciousness, patients on ventilators, and patients with severe dysphagia who have difficulty with oral nutrition.

4.2.4. Nutrition

Many people who develop pneumonia are under-nourished compared to those who do not develop pneumonia, and those who repeatedly develop pneumonia have difficulty getting enough calories and nutrients.

Nutritional intensification, calculated as the basal metabolism (Harris–Benedict formula) × physical activity coefficient (e.g., bed-ridden) × stress coefficient (1.1–1.2) using various nutritional routes, was intervened in bed-ridden elderly people for a period of one year [66]. Such an intervention not only reduced the number of pneumonia cases, but also improved other nutritional statuses (serum total protein and albumin levels) without the administration of albumin products. Thus, we re-iterate the need for nutritional treatment in order to help prevent pneumonia in the elderly.

A prospective cohort study considering a nutritional treatment intervention for the elderly at risk of pneumonia presented a significant reduction in morbidity related to pneumonia.

Furthermore, several nutrients are known to be associated with the development of pneumonia. Among other factors, the swallowing reflex is known to be depressed in patients with hypofolatemia below 3 ng/mL, as folic acid deficiency causes impaired metabolism of dopamine in the central nervous system. Supplementation with folic acid, accompanied by normalization of the plasma concentrations of homocysteine and folate, may improve the elicitation of the swallowing reflex [67].

Oral, tube (nasal tube feeding, gastrostomy), central venous, and peripheral venous nutrition nutritional options may be considered for patients who cannot receive adequate nutrition due to dysphagia. In a comparison of nutritional modalities, including oral, tube, and central venous nutrition options in bed-ridden elderly patients with dysphagia, tube feeding led to the longest survival (median, 23 months) [68]. Nutritional support by tube feeding reduces pneumonia-related morbidity and mortality, although it does not eliminate all cases of pneumonia, as compared with other means of nutrition or no nutritional support itself [69].

4.2.5. Swallowing Rehabilitation

While swallowing exercises such as the Mendelsohn manoeuvre, tongue-hold swallowing, supraglottal swallowing, shaker exercises, and effort pitch glide, as well as expiratory muscle strength training, have been shown to improve the structural excursion of each component, there have been no reports of reduced incidence of pneumonia with each exercise [70]. However, in a randomized control study of dysphagia patients with acute stroke, an intensive swallowing rehabilitation program using swallowing exercise therapy combined with a texture-modified diet showed a reduced incidence of under-nutrition and pneumonia [71]. Comprehensively, swallowing therapy including transcranial magnetic stimulation, transcranial direct current stimulation neuromuscular, electrical stimulation, and pharyngeal electrical stimulation has been reported to be effective in reducing the incidence of chest infection or pneumonia in the elderly with oropharyngeal dysphagia [72].

4.2.6. Oral Care

It is now common knowledge that oral care is effective in preventing the onset of pneumonia. In particular, an initial ground-breaking study, executed 20 years ago, showed that an oral care intervention for 2 years in institutionalized elderly people reduced the incidence of pneumonia in both dentulous and edentulous institutional elderly people [73]. Additionally, the cognitive function remained unchanged in the oral care intervention group compared to the non-intervention group. Further, in another one-month randomized controlled trial study conducted in a geriatric ward, the swallowing reflex latency shortened to a plateau after 10 days of oral care intervention, and the cough reflex sensitivity improved to the normal range after approximately one month [74,75]. In other words, oral care is not only about hygiene, but brushing itself can be considered a mechanical stimulus to gingival sensory nerve endings, and consequently to the central nervous system. Research reports have shown that nociception projects to the primary somatosensory cortex, as well as the cingulate and insular cortex (medial pain system), potentially supporting these results [76]. Furthermore, a one-year prospective cohort study of 343 nursing home residents has shown that residents with *Prevotella*, *Veillonella*, and *Treponema* spp. on their tongue coating, using a terminal restriction fragment length polymorphism (TRFLP) analysis, were pre-disposed to developing pneumonia [77]. Additionally, moisture retention on the tongue surfaces of those who developed pneumonia with these detected oral bacteria was low [77]. In other words, lower moisture retention may facilitate the growth of these bacteria associated with the development of pneumonia. Therefore, keeping the tongue moist with moisturising gel, together with oral brushing, may be expected to reduce the days of pyrexia and antimicrobial use, as well as the number of cases of pneumonia [78].

4.2.7. Sitting and Holding Position after Meals

AsP is most common in bed-ridden elderly patients. Many bed-ridden patients are unable to turn over on their own and lie in a supine position. Aspiration of the stomach contents, which can cause pneumonia, is less likely to occur in the semi-recumbent position than in the supine position [79,80]. Positions with a head angle of 30 degrees or more also reduce hospital-acquired pneumonia [81]. In bed-ridden institutionalized elderly patients, a 2 h post-prandial intervention in which the patients were placed at an angle of 30 degrees or more after a meal significantly reduced the number of fever days compared to the group without post-prandial intervention. Therefore, elderly people should be placed in a semi-recumbent position at 30° or higher for 2 h after eating [82]. A comparative study of positional changes showed that the semi-recumbent position reduced the frequency and risk of nosocomial pneumonia, especially in patients on enteral feeding [83].

Subsequently, the prone position has been advocated to prevent gastric reflux, inflammatory reactions, and alveolar over-expansion, as well as providing ventilation efficiency and oxygenation [84]. Therefore, in bed-ridden patients, the prone position may be more protective against the development of pneumonia than supine and even semi-recumbent positions.

4.2.8. Bowel Movement Control

Intestinal dysmotility is common in the elderly. Fecal impaction or stubborn constipation often leads to vomiting of gastrointestinal tract contents, resulting in the development of chemical pneumonitis. A high fiber content and moderate exercise are important for adequate control of bowel movements.

The gut–lung axis is not only physiological, but also involves microbial cross-talk [85]. Gut microbes in pulmonary host defence show that tonic signaling of pattern recognition receptors by microbial products in the steady state contributes to chronic lower respiratory diseases. Gut microbes act in the host's lung defence, and it has been reported that the tonic signal transduction when microbial products act on pattern recognition receptors contributes to chronic lower respiratory disease. High-fiber diets possibly increase the ratio of *Bacteroidetes* to *Firmicutes* species, and in consequence the production of short chain-fatty acids, which weaken the inflammation by activating GPR-40. It has been established that a high-fiber diet and short chain-fatty acids improve the intestinal microbial composition.

In clinical settings, most patients with recurrent AsP have difficulty eating sufficient fiber due to dysphagia, as well as having difficulty performing adequate exercise due to physical disability. Based on the above, the use of laxatives (as appropriate) may also be effective. Intervening with laxative medication in bed-ridden elderly patients without defecation for several days has been shown to reduce the incidence of pneumonitis but not pneumonia [28].

4.3. Strategies for Preventing Aspiration Pneumonia

Deterioration of the swallowing and coughing reflexes and low nutrition have been shown to be predictors of death within 90 days of AsP [46]. A disease time-axis for AsP and dysphagia has recently been identified (Figure 2). Therefore, to reduce the morbidity and mortality associated with AsP, priority should be given to improving the sensitivity of the swallowing reflex and cough reflex, as well as the nutritional status.

To begin, oral medicines are often difficult to administer to patients with dysphagia. Therefore, the following steps of resuming feeding and eating are recommended for patients at high risk of AsP. As a first step, during the acute fasting phase of antimicrobial treatment, aromatherapy intervention should be applied to activate the insular cortex, followed by a pureed or nectar-thickened meal containing capsaicin or menthol, in order to provoke both the swallowing reflex and cough reflex sensitivity levels. ACE-I, a dopamine-releasing agents, and phosphodiesterase-III inhibitors can be administered while gradually increasing the physicality of the meal. Oral care and swallowing rehabilitation should be consistently performed from the time of fasting. In our self-controlled case series, the intervention led to a significant decrease in the onset of pneumonia after the resumption of eating, which may indicate a certain effect (Figure 3) [86].

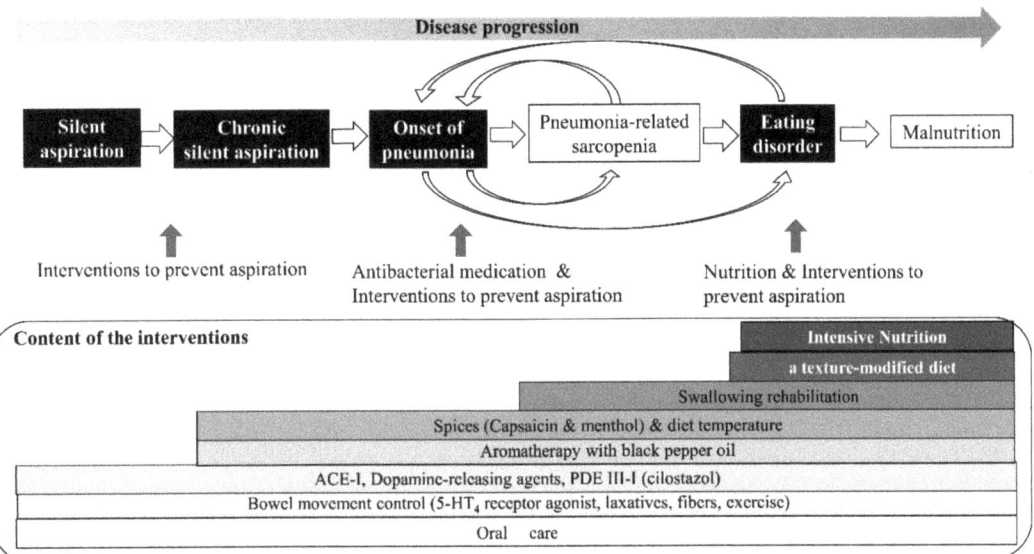

Figure 3. Disease time-axis and comprehensive approaches.

Additionally, when a patient is unable to intake sufficient calories and nutrients by mouth, it is recommended to provide essential nutrition through various nutritional routes, such as oral, gastrostomy, transcentral venous, or peripheral transvenous routes, with the step-wise eating and feeding methods mentioned above. This approach has the potential to reduce recurrent AsP and slow down the progression of dysphagia, thereby postponing the time to death. In clinical settings, we assume that while the state with inability to intake adequate nutrition orally stands as a gateway to the end of life for the elderly, there are many elderly individuals who may be able to escape from this gateway through nutritional support. Viewed another way, patients who have difficulties receiving essential nutrition due to diarrhoea during gastrostomy feeding, liver dysfunction, and repeated catheter-related bloodstream infections during central-venous nutrition may truly be at the end of their life.

5. Conclusions

There exists a pathophysiological time-axis of disease involving aspiration only, AsP, pneumonia-related sarcopenia, and eating disorders. Therefore, it is important to diagnose the position of an individuals on the disease time-axis in order to provide appropriate individualized treatment and prevention, taking into account their wishes and quality of life. Preventive measures to improve the upper airway reflex should be implemented from the disease onset to the end of life. Finally, education regarding how to prevent aspiration at home is important for both patients and their families and carers (see Table 1).

Table 1. How to prevent aspiration at home.

Before Eating
• Swallowing rehabilitation   • Aromatherapy (i.e., with black pepper oil)
Meals
• Spices (capsaicin and/or menthol)   • Diet temperature   • Texture-modified diet   • Fiber
After Eating
• Oral care   • A semi-recumbent position at 30° or higher for 2 h   • Laxatives (if appropriate)

Funding: This work was supported by the Japan Society for the Promotion of Science Grant-in-Aid for Scientific Research (C) KAKENHI (grant number 19152637) and by Japan Agency for Medical Research Science and Development (AMED) (grant number 17930474). The funders had no role in the study design, data collection and analysis, decision to publish, or preparation of the manuscript.

Institutional Review Board Statement: Not applicable due to narrative review.

Informed Consent Statement: Not applicable.

Data Availability Statement: The report did not report any data.

Conflicts of Interest: The authors declare no conflict of interest.

References

1. Lanspa, M.J.; Barbara, E.J.; Brown, S.M.; Dean, N.C. Mortality, morbidity, and disease severity of patients with aspiration pneumonia. *J. Hosp. Med.* **1996**, *8*, 83–90. [CrossRef] [PubMed]
2. Ministry of Health, Labour and Welfare, Japan. Available online: https://www.mhlw.go.jp/toukei/itiran/index.html (accessed on 1 March 2022).
3. Marik, P.E. Aspiration pneumonitis and aspiration pneumonia. *N. Engl. J. Med.* **2001**, *344*, 665–671. [CrossRef]
4. Baine, W.B.; Yu, W.; Summe, J.P. Epidemiologic trends in the hospitalization of elderly Medicare patients for pneumonia, 1991–1998. *Am. J. Public Health* **2001**, *91*, 1121–1123. [CrossRef] [PubMed]
5. Teramoto, S.; Fukuchi, Y.; Sasaki, H.; Sato, K.; Sekizawa, M.K.T.; Japanese Study Group on Aspiration Pulmonary Disease. High incidence of aspiration pneumonia in community- and hospital-acquired pneumonia in hospitalized patients: A multicenter, prospective study in Japan. *J. Am. Geriatr. Soc.* **2008**, *56*, 577–579. [CrossRef]
6. Yamaya, M.; Yanai, M.; Ohrui, T.; Arai, H.; Sasaki, H. Interventions to prevent pneumonia among older adults. *J. Am. Geriatr. Soc.* **2001**, *49*, 85–90. [CrossRef] [PubMed]
7. Lecci, A.; Giuliani, S.; Tramontana, M.; Carini, F.; Maggi, C.A. Peripheral actions of tachykinins. *Neuropeptides* **2000**, *34*, 303–313. [CrossRef]
8. Mutolo, D.; Bongianni, F.; Fontana, G.A.; Pantaleo, T. The role of excitatory amino acids and substance P in the mediation of the cough reflex within the nucleus tractus solitarii of the rabbit. *Brain Res. Bull.* **2007**, *74*, 284–293. [CrossRef] [PubMed]
9. Mutolo, D.; Bongianni, F.; Cinelli, E.; Pantaleo, T. Role of excitatory amino acids in the mediation of tracheobronchial cough induced by citric acid inhalation in the rabbit. *Brain Res. Bull.* **2009**, *80*, 22–29. [CrossRef] [PubMed]
10. Mazzone, S.B.; Mori, N.; Canning, B.J. Synergistic interactions between airway afferent nerve subtypes regulating the cough reflex in guinea pigs. *J. Physiol.* **2005**, *569*, 559–573. [CrossRef]
11. Ebihara, T.; Sekizawa, K.; Ohrui, T.; Nakazawa, H.; Sasaki, H. Angiotensin-converting enzyme inhibitor and danazol increase sensitivity of cough reflex in female guinea pigs. *Am. J. Respir Crit. Care Med.* **1996**, *153*, 812–819. [CrossRef] [PubMed]
12. Sekizawa, K.; Jia, Y.X.; Ebihara, T.; Hirose, Y.; Hirayama, Y.; Sasaki, H. Role of substance P in cough. *Pulm. Pharmacol.* **1996**, *9*, 323–328. [CrossRef] [PubMed]
13. Hope-Gill, B.D.M.; Hilldrup, S.; Davies, C.; Newton, R.P.; Harrison, N.K. A study of the cough reflex in idiopathic pulmonary fibrosis. *Am. J. Respir Crit Care Med.* **2003**, *168*, 995–1002. [CrossRef] [PubMed]
14. Sekizawa, K.; Ujiie, Y.; Itabashi, S.; Sasaki, H.; Takishima, T. Lack of cough reflex in aspiration pneumonia. *Lancet* **1990**, *335*, 1228–1229. [CrossRef]

15. Nakajoh, K.; Nakagawa, T.; Sekizawa, K.; Matsui, T.; Arai, H.; Sasaki, H. Relation between incidence of pneumonia and protective reflexes in post-stroke patients with oral or tube feeding. *J. Intern. Med.* **2000**, *247*, 39–42. [CrossRef] [PubMed]
16. Ebihara, T.; Sekizawa, K.; Nakazawa, H.; Sasaki, H. Capsaicin and swallowing reflex. *Lancet* **1993**, *341*, 432. [CrossRef]
17. Nakazawa, H.; Sekizawa, K.; Ujiie, Y.; Sasaki, H.; Takishima, T. Risk of aspiration pneumonia in the elderly. *Chest* **1993**, *103*, 1636–1637. [CrossRef]
18. Nakagawa, T.; Sekizawa, K.; Arai, H.; Kikuchi, R.; Manabe, K.; Sasaki, H. High incidence of pneumonia in elderly patients with basal ganglia infarction. *Arch. Intern. Med.* **1997**, *157*, 321–324. [CrossRef]
19. Jia, Y.X.; Sekizawa, K.; Ohrui, T.; Nakayama, K.; Sasaki, H. Dopamine D1 receptor antagonist inhibits swallowing reflex in guinea pigs. *Am. J. Physiol.* **1998**, *274*, R76–R80. [CrossRef]
20. Okamura, N.; Maruyama, M.; Ebihara, T.; Matsui, T.; Nemoto, M.; Arai, H.; Sasaki, H.; Yanai, K. Aspiration pneumonia and insular hypoperfusion in patients with cerebrovascular disease. *J. Am. Geriatr. Soc.* **2004**, *52*, 645–646. [CrossRef]
21. Humbert, I.A.; Robbins, J. Normal swallowing and functional magnetic resonance imaging: A systematic review. *Dysphagia* **2007**, *22*, 266–275. [CrossRef]
22. Suzuki, M.; Asada, Y.; Ito, J.; Hayashi, K.; Inoue, H.; Kitano, H. Activation of cerebellum and basal ganglia on volitional swallowing detected by functional magnetic resonance imaging. *Dysphagia* **2003**, *18*, 71–77. [CrossRef] [PubMed]
23. Hamdy, S.; Rothwell, J.C.; Aziz, Q.; Singh, K.D.; Thompson, D.G. Long-term reorganization of human motor cortex driven by short-term sensory stimulation. *Nat. Neurosci.* **1998**, *1*, 64–68. [CrossRef]
24. Anderson, T.M.; Garcia, A.J.; Baertsch, N.A.; Pollak, J.; Bloom, J.C.; Wei, A.D.; Rai, K.G.; Ramirez, J.M. A novel excitatory network for the control of breathing. *Nature* **2016**, *536*, 76–80. [CrossRef] [PubMed]
25. Yagi, N.; Oku, Y.; Nagami, S.; Yamagata, Y.; Kayashita, J.; Ishikawa, A.; Domen, K.; Takahashi, R. Inappropriate timing of swallow in the respiratory cycle causes breathing-swallowing discoordination. *Front. Physiol.* **2017**, *22*, 676. [CrossRef] [PubMed]
26. Marumo, K.; Homma, S.; Fukuchi, Y. Postgastrectomy aspiration pneumonia. *Chest* **1995**, *107*, 453–456. [CrossRef] [PubMed]
27. Ebihara, T.; Ebihara, S.; Ida, S.; Ohrui, T.; Yasuda, H.; Sasaki, H.; Arai, H. Acid and swallowing reflex. *Geriatr. Gerontol. Int.* **2007**, *7*, 94–95. [CrossRef]
28. Fujii, M.; Sasaki, H. Constipation and aspiration pneumonia. *Geriatr. Gerontol. Int.* **2012**, *12*, 570–571. [CrossRef]
29. Nagamine, T. Serum substance P levels in patients with chronic schizophrenia treated with typical or atypical antipsychotics. *Neuropsychiatr. Dis. Treat.* **2008**, *4*, 289–294. [CrossRef]
30. Herzig, S.J.; LaSalvia, M.T.; Naidus, E.; Rothberg, M.B.; Zhou, W.; Gurwitz, J.H.; Marcantonio, E.R. Antipsychotics and the risk of aspiration pneumonia in individuals hospitalized for nonpsychiatric conditions: A cohort study. *J. Am. Geriatr. Soc.* **2017**, *65*, 2580–2586. [CrossRef]
31. Kose, E.; Hirai, T.; Seki, T. Assessment of aspiration pneumonia using the anticholinergic risk scale. *Geriatr. Gerontol. Int.* **2018**, *18*, 1230–1235. [CrossRef]
32. Marchina, S.; Doros, G.; Modak, J.; Helenius, J.; Aycock, D.M.; Kumar, S. Acid-suppressive medications and risk of pneumonia in acute stroke patients: A systematic review and meta-analysis. *J. Neurol. Sci.* **2019**, *400*, 122–128. [CrossRef] [PubMed]
33. Tranberg, A.; Samuelsson, C.; Klarin, B. Disturbance in the oropharyngeal microbiota in relation to antibiotic and proton pump inhibitor medication and length of hospital stay. *APMIS* **2021**, *129*, 14–22. [CrossRef] [PubMed]
34. Morley, J.E.; Baumgartner, R.N.; Roubenoff, R.; Mayer, J.; Nair, K.S. Sarcopenia. *J. Lab. Clin. Med.* **2001**, *137*, 231–243. [CrossRef] [PubMed]
35. Giordano, C.; Lemaire, C.; Li, T.; Kimoff, R.J.; Petrof, B.J. Autophagy-associated atrophy and metabolic remodeling of the mouse diaphragm after short-term intermittent hypoxia. *PLoS ONE* **2015**, *24*, e0131068. [CrossRef] [PubMed]
36. Altuna-Venegas, S.; Aliaga-Vega, R.; Maguiña, J.L.; Parodi, J.F.; Runzer-Colmenares, F.M. Risk of community-acquired pneumonia in older adults with sarcopenia of a hospital from Callao, Peru 2010–2015. *Arch. Gerontol. Geriatr.* **2019**, *82*, 100–105. [CrossRef] [PubMed]
37. Okazaki, T.; Liang, F.; Li, T.; Danialou, G.; Shoelson, S.E.; Petrof, B.J. Muscle-specific inhibition of the classical nuclear factor-κB pathway is protective against diaphragmatic weakness in murine endotoxemia. *Crit. Care Med.* **2014**, *42*, e501–e509. [CrossRef] [PubMed]
38. Looijaard, W.G.P.M.; Dekker, I.M.; Beishuizen, A.; Girbes, A.R.J.; Oudemans-van Straaten, H.M.; Weijs, P.J.M. Early high protein intake and mortality in critically ill ICU patients with low skeletal muscle area and density. *Clin. Nutr.* **2020**, *39*, 2192–2201. [CrossRef]
39. Okazaki, T.; Ebihara, S.; Mori, T.; Izumi, S.; Ebihara, T. Association between sarcopenia and pneumonia in older people. *Rev. Geriatr. Gerontol. Int.* **2020**, *20*, 7–13. [CrossRef]
40. Okazaki, T.; Suzukamo, Y.; Miyatake, M.; Komatsu, R.; Yaekashiwa, M.; Nihei, M.; Izumi, S.; Ebihara, T. Respiratory muscle weakness as a risk factor for pneumonia in older people. *Gerontology* **2021**, *67*, 581–590. [CrossRef]
41. Shiozu, H.; Higashijima, M.; Koga, T. Association of sarcopenia with swallowing problems, related to nutrition and activities of daily living of elderly individuals. *J. Phys. Sci.* **2015**, *27*, 393–396. [CrossRef]
42. Murakami, M.; Hirano, H.; Watanabe, Y.; Sakai, K.; Kim, H.; Katakura, A. Relationship between chewing ability and sarcopenia in Japanese community-dwelling older adults. *Geriatr. Gerontol. Int.* **2015**, *15*, 1007–1012. [CrossRef]
43. Kuroda, Y.; Kuroda, R. Relationship between thinness and swallowing function in Japanese older adults: Implications for sarcopenic dysphagia. *J. Am. Geriatr. Soc.* **2012**, *60*, 1785–1786, Erratum in: *J. Am. Geriatr. Soc.* **2012**, *60*, 2385. [CrossRef]

44. Ogawa, N.; Mori, T.; Fujishima, I.; Wakabayashi, H.; Itoda, M.; Kunieda, K.; Shigematsu, T.; Nishioka, S.; Tohara, H.; Yamada, M.; et al. Ultrasonography to measure swallowing muscle mass and quality in older patients with sarcopenic dysphagia. *J. Am. Med. Dir. Assoc.* **2018**, *19*, 516–522. [CrossRef] [PubMed]
45. Maeda, K.; Akagi, J. Decreased tongue pressure is associated with sarcopenia and sarcopenic dysphagia in the elderly. *Dysphagia* **2015**, *30*, 80–87, Erratum in: *Dysphagia* 2015, 30, 88. [CrossRef] [PubMed]
46. Ebihara, T.; Miyamoto, T.; Kozaki, K. Prognostic factors of 90-day mortality in older people with healthcare-associated pneumonia. *Geriatr. Gerontol. Int.* **2020**, *20*, 1036–1043. [CrossRef]
47. Miyamoto, T.; Ebihara, T.; Kozaki, K. The association between eating difficulties and biliary sludge in the gallbladder in older adults with advanced dementia, at end of life. *PLoS ONE* **2019**, *14*, e0219538. [CrossRef] [PubMed]
48. Dicpinigaitis, P.V. Angiotensin-converting enzyme inhibitor-induced cough: ACCP evidence-based clinical practice guidelines. *Chest* **2006**, *129*, 169S–173S. [CrossRef] [PubMed]
49. Tomaki, M.; Ichinose, M.; Miura, M.; Hirayama, Y.; Kageyama, N.; Yamauchi, H.; Shirato, K. Angiotensin converting enzyme (ACE) inhibitor-induced cough and substance P. *Thorax* **1996**, *51*, 199–201. [CrossRef]
50. Nakayama, K.; Sekizawa, K.; Sasaki, H. ACE inhibitor and swallowing reflex. *Chest* **1998**, *113*, 1425. [CrossRef]
51. Sekizawa, K.; Matsui, T.; Nakagawa, T.; Nakayama, K.; Sasaki, H. ACE inhibitors and pneumonia. *Lancet* **1998**, *352*, 1069. [CrossRef]
52. Arai, T.; Sekizawa, K.; Ohrui, T.; Fujiwara, H.; Yoshimi, N.; Matsuoka, H.; Sasaki, H. ACE inhibitors and protection against pneumonia in elderly patients with stroke. *Neurology* **2005**, *64*, 573–574. [CrossRef] [PubMed]
53. Nakagawa, T.; Wada, H.; Sekizawa, K.; Arai, H.; Sasaki, H. Amantadine and pneumonia. *Lancet* **1999**, *353*, 1157. [CrossRef]
54. Kanda, A.; Ebihara, S.; Yasuda, H.; Takashi, O.; Sasaki, T.; Sasaki, H. A combinatorial therapy for pneumonia in elderly people. *J. Am. Geriatr. Soc.* **2004**, *52*, 846–847. [CrossRef] [PubMed]
55. Yamaguchi, H.; Maki, Y.; Maki, Y. Tube feeding can be discontinued by taking dopamine agonists and angiotensin-converting enzyme inhibitors in the advanced stages of dementia. *J. Am. Geriatr. Soc.* **2010**, *58*, 2035–2036. [CrossRef] [PubMed]
56. Yamaya, M.; Yanai, M.; Ohrui, T.; Arai, H.; Sekizawa, K.; Sasaki, H. Antithrombotic therapy for prevention of pneumonia. *J. Am. Geriatr. Soc.* **2001**, *49*, 687–688. [CrossRef] [PubMed]
57. Netsu, S.; Mizuma, A.; Sakamoto, M.; Yutani, S.; Nagata, E.; Takizawaet, S. Cilostazol is effective to prevent stroke-associated pneumonia in patients receiving tube feeding. *Dysphagia* **2018**, *33*, 716–724. [CrossRef] [PubMed]
58. Osawa, A.; Maeshima, S.; Tanahashi, N. Efficacy of cilostazol in preventing aspiration pneumonia in acute cerebral infarction. *J. Stroke Cereb. Dis.* **2013**, *22*, 857–861. [CrossRef] [PubMed]
59. He, M.; Ohrui, T.; Ebihara, T.; Ebihara, S.; Sasaki, H.; Arai, H. Mosapride citrate prolongs survival in stroke patients with gastrostomy. *J. Am. Geriatr. Soc.* **2007**, *55*, 142–144. [CrossRef] [PubMed]
60. Takatori, K.; Yoshida, R.; Horai, A.; Satake, S.; Ose, T.; Kitajima, N.; Yoneda, S.; Adachi, K.; Amano, Y.; Kinoshita, Y. Therapeutic effects of mosapride citrate and lansoprazole for prevention of aspiration pneumonia in patients receiving gastrostomy feeding. *J. Gastroenterol.* **2013**, *48*, 1105–1110. [CrossRef]
61. Hamlet, S.; Choi, J.; Zormeier, M.; Shamsa, F.; Stachler, R.; Muz, J.; Jones, L. Normal adult swallowing of liquid and viscous material: Scintigraphic data on bolus transit and oropharyngeal residues. *Dysphagia* **1996**, *11*, 41–47. [CrossRef]
62. Beck, A.M.; Kjaersgaard, A.; Hansen, T.; Poulsen, I. Systematic review and evidence-based recommendations on texture modified foods and thickened liquids for adults (above 17 years) with oropharyngeal dysphagia—An updated clinical guideline. *Clin. Nutr.* **2018**, *37*, 1980–1991. [CrossRef]
63. Watando, A.; Ebihara, S.; Ebihara, T.; Okazaki, T.; Takahashi, H.; Asada, M.; Sasaki, H. Effect of temperature on swallowing reflex in elderly patients with aspiration pneumonia. *J. Am. Geriatr. Soc.* **2004**, *52*, 2143–2144. [CrossRef] [PubMed]
64. Ebihara, T.; Ebihara, S.; Watando, A.; Okazaki, T.; Asada, M.; Ohrui, T.; Yamaya, M.; Arai, H. Effects of menthol on the triggering of the swallowing reflex in elderly patients with dysphagia. *Br. J. Clin. Pharmacol.* **2006**, *62*, 369–371. [CrossRef] [PubMed]
65. Ebihara, T.; Yamasaki, M.; Kozaki, K.; Ebihara, S. Medical aromatherapy in geriatric syndrome. *Geriatr. Gerontol. Int.* **2021**, *21*, 377–385. [CrossRef] [PubMed]
66. Yamaya, M.; Kawakami, G.; Momma, H.; Yamada, A.; Itoh, J.; Ichinose, M. Effects of Nutritional Treatment on the Frequency of Pneumonia in Bedridden Patients Receiving Oral Care. *Intern. Med.* **2020**, *59*, 181–192. [CrossRef]
67. Sato, E.; Ohrui, T.; Matsui, T.; Arai, H.; Sasaki, H. Folate deficiency and risk of pneumonia in older people. *J. Am. Geriatr. Soc.* **2001**, *49*, 1739–1740. [CrossRef]
68. Kosaka, Y.; Yamaya, M.; Nakajoh, K.; Matsui, T.; Yanai, M.; Sasaki, H. Prognosis of elderly patients with dysphagia in Japan. *Gerontology* **2000**, *46*, 111–112. [CrossRef] [PubMed]
69. Kosaka, Y.; Nakagawa-Satoh, T.; Ohrui, T.; Fujii, M.; Arai, H.; Sasaki, H. Survival period after tube feeding in bedridden older patients. *Geriatr. Gerontol. Int.* **2012**, *12*, 317–321. [CrossRef] [PubMed]
70. Balou, M.; Herzberg, E.G.; Kamelhar, D.; Molfenter, S.M. An intensive swallowing exercise protocol for improving swallowing physiology in older adults with radiographically confirmed dysphagia. *Clin. Interv. Aging* **2019**, *11*, 283–288. [CrossRef]
71. Carnaby, G.; Hankey, G.J.; Pizzi, J. Behavioural intervention for dysphagia in acute stroke: A randomised controlled trial. *Lancet Neurol.* **2006**, *5*, 31–37. [CrossRef]
72. Bath, P.M.; Lee, H.S.; Everton, L.F. Swallowing therapy for dysphagia in acute and subacute stroke. *Cochrane Database Syst. Rev.* **2018**, *10*, CD000323. [CrossRef] [PubMed]

73. Yoneyama, T.; Yoshida, M.; Ohrui, T.; Mukaiyama, H.; Okamoto, H.; Hoshiba, K.; Ihara, S.; Yanagisawa, S.; Ariumi, S.; Morita, T.; et al. Oral Care Working Group. Oral care reduces pneumonia in older patients in nursing homes. *J. Am. Geriatr. Soc.* **2002**, *50*, 430–433. [CrossRef] [PubMed]
74. Yoshino, A.; Ebihara, T.; Ebihara, S.; Fuji, H.; Sasaki, H. Daily oral care and risk factors for pneumonia among elderly nursing home patients. *JAMA* **2001**, *286*, 2235–2236. [CrossRef]
75. Watando, A.; Ebihara, S.; Ebihara, T.; Okazaki, T.; Takahashi, H.; Asada, M.; Sasaki, H. Daily oral care and cough reflex sensitivity in elderly nursing home patients. *Chest* **2004**, *126*, 1066–1070. [CrossRef] [PubMed]
76. Weigelt, A.; Terekhin, P.; Kemppainen, P.; Dörfler, A.; Forster, C. The representation of experimental tooth pain from upper and lower jaws in the human trigeminal pathway. *Pain* **2010**, *149*, 529–538. [CrossRef]
77. Takeshita, T.; Tomioka, M.; Shimazaki, Y.; Matsuyama, M.; Koyano, K.; Matsuda, K.; Yamashita, Y. Microfloral characterization of the tongue coating and associated risk for pneumonia-related health problems in institutionalized older adults. *J. Am. Geriatr. Soc.* **2010**, *58*, 1050–1057. [CrossRef] [PubMed]
78. Sudo, E.; Maejima, I. The effects of moisturizing gel to prevent dry mouth in patients with cerebrovascular disease. *Nihon. Ronen Igakkai. Zasshi.* **2008**, *45*, 196–201. (In Japanese) [CrossRef]
79. Torres, A.; Serra-Batlles, J.; Ros, E.; Piera, C.; de la Bellacasa, J.P.; Cobos, A.; Lomeña, F.; Rodríguez-Roisin, R. Pulmonary aspiration of gastric contents in patients receiving mechanical ventilation: The effect of body position. *Ann. Intern. Med.* **1992**, *116*, 540–543. [CrossRef] [PubMed]
80. Orozco-Levi, M.; Torres, A.; Ferrer, M.; Piera, C.; el-Ebiary, M.; de la Bellacasa, J.P.; Rodriguez-Roisin, R. Semi-recumbent position protects from pulmonary aspiration but not completely from gastroesophageal reflux in mechanically ventilated patients. *Am. J. Respir. Crit. Care Med.* **1995**, *152*, 1387–1390. [CrossRef]
81. Fernández-Crehuet, R.; Díaz-Molina, C.; de Irala, J.; Martínez-Concha, D.; Salcedo-Leal, I.; Masa-Calles, J. Nosocomial infection in an intensive-care unit: Identification of risk factors. *Infect. Control Hosp. Epidemiol.* **1997**, *18*, 825–830. [PubMed]
82. Matsui, T.; Yamaya, M.; Ohrui, T.; Arai, H.; Sasaki, H. Sitting position to prevent aspiration in bed-bound patients. *Gerontology* **2002**, *48*, 194–195. [CrossRef] [PubMed]
83. Drakulovic, M.B.; Torres, A.; Bauer, T.T.; Nicolas, J.M.; Nogué, S.; Ferrer, M. Supine body position as a risk factor for nosocomial pneumonia in mechanically ventilated patients: A randomized trial. *Lancet* **1999**, *354*, 1851–1858. [CrossRef]
84. Galiatsou, E.; Kostanti, E.; Svarna, E.; Kitsakos, A.; Koulouras, V.; Efremidis, S.C.; Nakos, G. Prone position augments recruitment and prevents alveolar overinflation in acute lung injury. *Am. J. Respir. Crit. Care Med.* **2006**, *174*, 187–197. [CrossRef] [PubMed]
85. Dang, A.T.; Marsland, B.J. Microbes, metabolites, and the gut-lung axis. *Mucosal Immunol.* **2019**, *12*, 843–850. [CrossRef]
86. Ebihara, T.; Ebihara, S.; Yamazaki, M.; Asada, M.; Yamanda, S.; Arai, H. Intensive stepwise method for oral intake using a combination of transient receptor potential stimulation and olfactory stimulation inhibits the incidence of pneumonia in dysphagic older adults. *J. Am. Geriatr. Soc.* **2010**, *58*, 196–198. [CrossRef] [PubMed]

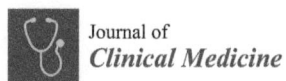

Article

High Mortality in an Older Japanese Population with Low Forced Vital Capacity and Gender-Dependent Potential Impact of Muscle Strength: Longitudinal Cohort Study

Midori Miyatake [1], Tatsuma Okazaki [1,2,*], Yoshimi Suzukamo [1], Sanae Matsuyama [3], Ichiro Tsuji [3] and Shin-Ichi Izumi [1,2,4]

1. Department of Physical Medicine and Rehabilitation, Tohoku University Graduate School of Medicine, Sendai 980-8575, Japan
2. Center for Dysphagia of Tohoku University Hospital, Sendai 980-8575, Japan
3. Division of Epidemiology, Department of Health Informatics and Public Health, School of Public Health, Tohoku University Graduate School of Medicine, Sendai 980-8575, Japan
4. Department of Physical Medicine and Rehabilitation, Tohoku University Graduate School of Biomedical Engineering, Sendai 980-8575, Japan
* Correspondence: tmokazaki0808@gmail.com; Tel.: +81-22-717-7338

Abstract: Generally, weak muscle power is associated with high mortality. We aimed to evaluate the unknown association between % predicted value forced vital capacity (FVC% predicted) and mortality in asymptomatic older people, and the impact of muscle power on this association. We analyzed the Tsurugaya cohort that enrolled Japanese people aged ≥70 for 15 years with Cox proportional hazards model. Exposure variables were FVC% predicted and leg power. The outcome was all-cause mortality. The subjects were divided into quartiles by FVC% predicted or leg power, or into two groups by 80% for FVC% predicted or by the strongest 25% for leg power. Across 985 subjects, 262 died. The males with lower FVC% predicted exhibited higher mortality risks. The hazard ratio (HR) was 2.03 (95% CI 1.30–3.18) at the lowest relative to the highest groups. The addition of leg power reduced the HR to 1.78 (95% CI 1.12–2.80). In females, FVC% predicted under 80% was a risk factor and the HR was 1.67 (95% CI 1.05–2.64) without the effect of leg power. In FVC% predicted <80% males HRs were 2.44 (95% CI 1.48–4.02) in weak and 1.38 (95% CI 0.52–3.64) in strong leg power males, relative to ≥80% and strong leg power males. Low FVC% predicted was associated with high mortality with potential unfavorable effects of weak leg power in males.

Keywords: % predicted value forced vital capacity; mortality; muscle strength; older people; cohort study; pneumonia

Citation: Miyatake, M.; Okazaki, T.; Suzukamo, Y.; Matsuyama, S.; Tsuji, I.; Izumi, S.-I. High Mortality in an Older Japanese Population with Low Forced Vital Capacity and Gender-Dependent Potential Impact of Muscle Strength: Longitudinal Cohort Study. *J. Clin. Med.* **2022**, *11*, 5264. https://doi.org/10.3390/jcm11185264

Academic Editors: Enrico M. Clini and Satoru Ebihara

Received: 20 July 2022
Accepted: 2 September 2022
Published: 6 September 2022

Publisher's Note: MDPI stays neutral with regard to jurisdictional claims in published maps and institutional affiliations.

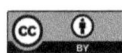

Copyright: © 2022 by the authors. Licensee MDPI, Basel, Switzerland. This article is an open access article distributed under the terms and conditions of the Creative Commons Attribution (CC BY) license (https://creativecommons.org/licenses/by/4.0/).

1. Introduction

Forced vital capacity (FVC) and % predicted value FVC (FVC% predicted) are major indicators of respiratory functions. Several general population studies reported an association between low FVC/FVC% predicted and high mortality [1–6]. FVC and FVC% predicted are generally used to diagnose restrictive lung diseases, typically represented by interstitial lung diseases. Patients with interstitial lung diseases are accompanied by high mortality [7,8]. A previous study avoided the effects of interstitial lung diseases on mortality by excluding people with respiratory symptoms and showed an association between low FVC and high mortality in general adults [9]. However, another study that analyzed older people with a rather short follow-up period could not show an association [10]. Presently, we only have limited information about the association between FVC% predicted and long-term mortality in community-dwelling older people without respiratory symptoms.

Many studies reported an association between extremity muscle weakness and high mortality [11–16]. Extremity muscle strength and respiratory function are moderately correlated with respiratory muscle strength [17–20]. Respiratory muscle weakness is associated with the onset of and potentially death by pneumonia in older people [21]. Presently, the effects of muscle strength on the association between FVC% predicted and mortality are unclear.

The main objective of this study was to investigate the association between low FVC% predicted and high mortality in community-dwelling asymptomatic older people. Our secondary objective was to determine whether weak extremity muscle power has an unfavorable effect on the association between low FVC% predicted and high mortality. We hypothesized that low FVC% predicted was associated with high mortality in general asymptomatic older people. We next hypothesized that extremity muscle weakness has an unfavorable effect on the association. To achieve the above objectives, we analyzed a longitudinal cohort, the Tsurugaya project.

2. Materials and Methods

2.1. Participants

We used the baseline data from 2002 on the comprehensive geriatric assessments conducted for older people aged ≥70 years in the Tsurugaya project [22,23]. We excluded potential interstitial lung disease patients by evaluating dyspnea as a respiratory symptom. Dyspnea was evaluated by breathing through an external circuit with an inspiratory resistive load of 10, 20, and 30 $cmH_2O/L/s$ and was assessed by the modified Borg scale [24,25]. This is a category scale in which the subject selects a number from 0 (no dyspnea) to 10 (maximum dyspnea). Subjects selected 2 or greater at baseline breathing without inspiratory resistance for 1 minute were excluded.

2.2. Measurements

Spirometry (OST 80A, Chest Co., Tokyo, Japan) was measured 3 times, and the best trial was reported. The FVC% predicted values were calculated by age, gender, and height [26]. Initial measurements were performed in 2002, following American Thoracic Society recommendations [27], applying reference values and a cut-off value for FVC as 80% to FVC% predicted, as the Japanese respiratory society published in 2001. Current Japanese reference values were published in 2014; however, we applied the old reference values in this study to keep consistency within the Tsurugaya project [24,26]. In each gender, the subjects were divided into 4 groups based on quartiles of FVC% predicted or 2 groups (<80% and ≥80%) [26]. Leg extension power (w/kg) was measured on a horizontal leg extension apparatus (Combi Anaeropress3500, Tokyo, Japan) [28]. The average of the 2 strongest leg power measurements among 5 trials was divided by the bodyweight [28]. In each gender, the subjects were divided into 4 groups based on quartiles or into 2 groups, the strongest 25% group and other groups. Sociodemographic and medical history data were collected using questionnaires. The questionnaire included age, sex, medical history (pneumonia, bronchial asthma, cancer, myocardial infarction, stroke, diabetes, hypertension), smoking, alcohol consumption, educational levels, and marital status. The smoking status and alcohol consumption were categorical variables; subjects were classified into current, past, or never smoking groups and non-alcohol, current, or past consumption groups. The educational periods categorized the subjects into <18- or ≥18-year groups. Depressive symptoms were evaluated with the Japanese version of the 30-point Geriatric Depression Scale (GDS) [29], and cognitive function was measured with the Japanese version of the Mini-Mental State Examination (MMSE) [30]. The serum albumin and high sensitive C-reactive protein (hs-CRP) concentrations were assessed in blood samples collected under non-fasting conditions by a clinical testing laboratory. Body mass index (BMI, kg/m^2) was calculated.

2.3. Mortality Follow-Up

The outcome of the study was all-cause mortality. Data regarding death or migration were received from the Sendai Municipal Authority. The follow-up period was from 30 March 2003 to 1 July 2018.

2.4. Statistical Analysis

The baseline characteristics of 4 groups divided by FVC% predicted were compared by chi-square tests for categorical variables and one-way ANOVA for continuous variables. The cumulative survival rate of the 4 groups was compared according to the FVC% predicted using the Kaplan–Meier method and log-rank tests. The Cox proportional hazard model was used to calculate the hazard ratios (HRs) and 95% confidence intervals (CIs) for all-cause mortality during the follow-up period. The highest group was used as the reference category. To investigate the relationships among the 4 groups for FVC% predicted and all-cause mortality, we ran 2 models. Model 1 was a univariate model. Model 2 was adjusted by all potential covariates; potential covariates for adjustment included age, medical histories (pneumonia, bronchial asthma, cancer, stroke, myocardial infarction, diabetes, hypertension), smoking, alcohol consumption, depressive symptoms, cognitive function, educational level, marital status, leg power (divided into 4 groups), BMI, albumin, and hs-CRP. The 1 and 2 models were also applied to investigate the relationship between the 2 groups for FVC% predicted divided by the clinical cut-off value of $\geq$80% and all-cause mortality. We also evaluated the effect of muscle strength (divided into 4 groups) on the relationship among the 4 groups for FVC% predicted and all-cause mortality. Model 1 was a univariate model. Leg power was added as an explanatory variable in Model 2. Model 3 was adjusted by all potential covariates. The 1–3 models were also applied to investigate the effect of muscle strength divided by the strongest 25% on the relationship between FVC% predicted divided by $\geq$80% and all-cause mortality. To evaluate the relationship between muscle strength, FVC% predicted, and mortality, we divided the subjects into 2 groups by $\geq$80% for FVC% predicted and by the strongest 25% for muscle strength, respectively, a total of 4 groups. Model 1 was a univariate model. Model 2 was adjusted by all potential covariates. We also conducted a sensitivity analysis to test the robustness of the association between FVC% predicted and all-cause mortality. The above statistical analyses were performed using SPSS software, version 24.0 (IBM Corp., Armonk, NY, USA). We evaluated the power of the main result by the post hoc power analysis using Power and Precision 4.1 (Biostat, Englewood, NJ, USA). p values less than 0.05 were considered significant.

3. Results

We invited all residents who were $\geq$70 years old to the Tsurugaya project in 2002 (n = 2730). Of 1198 participating subjects, 1175 provided written informed consent. Figure 1 shows a study flow chart. Nineteen subjects without spirometry data and 95 subjects with missing or incomplete leg extension power data were excluded. We excluded eight subjects with a Mini-Mental State Examination (MMSE) score below 10 or missing to maintain the reliability of the spirometry data. Nineteen subjects lacked high-sensitive C-reactive protein (hs-CRP) data. We excluded 49 subjects with respiratory symptoms to exclude potential interstitial lung disease patients. Finally, 985 subjects were analyzed.

The subjects were divided by gender and then into four groups by FVC% predicted (Quartile1: FVC% predicted $\geq$100.5 [male], $\geq$114.5 [female]; Quartile2: $\geq$89.2 to <100.5 [male], $\geq$100.9 to <114.5 [female]; Quartile3: $\geq$78.3 to <89.2 [male], $\geq$87.7 to <100.9 [female]; and Quartile4: <78.3 [male], <87.7 [female]). Quartile 1 was the highest and Quartile 4 was the lowest FVC% predicted group. Table 1 shows the characteristics recorded in the baseline survey. Among the 985 participants, the proportion of males was 42.6%, and the mean age (standard deviation [SD]) was 75.6 (4.8) years. The variables that showed significant differences among the four groups were age, education levels, the incidence of past histories of pneumonia and bronchial asthma, leg extension power, and hs-CRP.

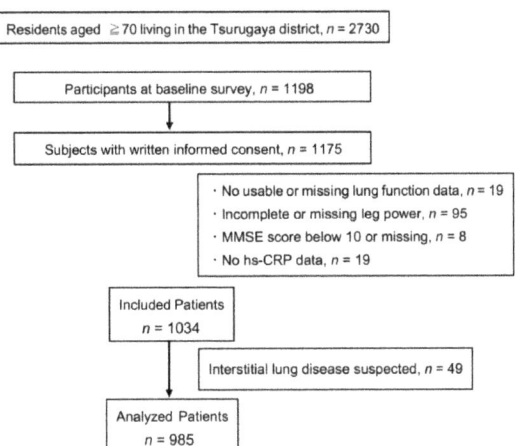

Figure 1. Inclusion and exclusion of the study participants. MMSE = Mini-Mental State Examination, hs-CRP = high-sensitive C-reactive protein.

Table 1. Baseline characteristics of the study participants according to FVC% predicted ($n = 985$).

Characteristics	FVC% Predicted					
	Overall	Q1 ‡	Q2 §	Q3 ‖	Q4 **	p *
Number of participants	985	246	247	247	245	
Age, mean (SD)	75.6 (4.8)	75.9 (5.2)	75.4 (4.7)	75.1 (4.2)	76.1 (4.8)	0.047
Men, n (%)	420 (42.6)	105 (42.7)	105 (42.5)	106 (42.9)	104 (42.4)	1.000
Medical history, n (%)						
Pneumonia	92 (9.3)	17 (6.9)	23 (9.3)	16 (6.5)	36 (14.7)	0.006
Bronchial asthma	56 (6.0)	8 (3.3)	10 (4.0)	14 (5.7)	27 (11.0)	0.001
Cancer	65 (6.6)	18 (7.3)	15 (6.1)	18 (7.3)	14 (5.7)	0.845
Myocardial infarction	108 (11.0)	24 (9.8)	29 (11.7)	29 (11.7)	26 (10.6)	0.872
Stroke	46 (4.7)	15 (6.1)	9 (3.6)	14 (5.7)	8 (3.3)	0.341
Diabetes mellitus	138 (14.0)	39 (15.9)	33 (13.4)	29 (11.7)	37 (15.1)	0.556
Hypertension	370 (37.6)	77 (31.3)	94 (38.1)	98 (39.7)	101 (41.2)	0.111
Current smoking, n (%)	130 (13.2)	33 (13.7)	32 (13.2)	30 (12.4)	35 (14.7)	0.924
Alcohol consumption, n (%)	400 (40.6)	107 (45.5)	100 (42.4)	109 (46.6)	84 (36.4)	0.174
Duration of education ≥18 years, n (%) †	561 (57.0)	143 (58.4)	145 (58.9)	153 (62.2)	120 (49.6)	0.034
Marital status, n (%)	609 (61.8)	156 (63.4)	157 (63.6)	147 (59.5)	149 (61.6)	0.950
Cognitive impairment, mean (SD)	27.4 (2.6)	27.5 (2.5)	27.6 (2.3)	27.2 (2.8)	27.1 (2.8)	0.067
Depressive symptoms, mean (SD)	8.9 (5.4)	8.6 (5.4)	9.0 (5.6)	8.7 (5.6)	9.2 (5.0)	0.553
BMI (kg/m^2), mean (SD)	23.8 (3.3)	23.5 (3.0)	23.8 (3.1)	24.1 (3.2)	23.7 (3.8)	0.135
Leg extension power (w/kg), mean (SD)	10.1 (4.5)	10.8 (4.8)	10.4 (4.4)	9.9 (4.5)	9.0 (4.1)	<0.001
Albumin, (g/dL), mean (SD)	4.3 (0.3)	4.3 (0.3)	4.3 (0.3)	4.3 (0.3)	4.3 (0.3)	0.634
hs-CRP (ng/mL), mean (SD)	1790 (5325)	965 (1581)	2068 (7276)	1563 (4459)	2565 (6084)	<0.001

FVC% predicted = % predicted value forced vital capacity; SD = standard deviation; BMI = body mass index; hs-CRP = high sensitive C-reactive protein; ANOVA = analysis of variance. * Obtained by using chi-squared test for variables of proportion and one-factor ANOVA for continuous variables. † Age at last school graduation 18 years. ‡ Q1; FVC% predicted ≥100.5 (male), ≥114.5 (female). § Q2; FVC% predicted ≥89.2 to <100.5 (male), ≥100.9 to <114.5 (female). ‖ Q3; FVC% predicted ≥78.3 to <89.2 (male), ≥87.7 to <100.9 (female). ** Q4; FVC% predicted <78.3 (male), <87.7 (female).

During the follow-up period of 13,011 person-years, of the 420 males, 154 (36.7%) died, and of the 565 females, 108 (19.1%) died. Figure 2 shows Kaplan–Meier survival curves according to the FVC% predicted in males (Figure 2A) and females (Figure 2B). The cumulative survival rates were significantly lower in the lowest FVC% predicted group Quartile 4 in males (log-rank test, $p < 0.005$), but there were no differences in females (log-rank test, $p = 0.193$). The number at risk in Figure 2 showed the number of individuals at risk of experiencing an event for each cohort during the follow-up period every 2 years. Figure 2 also showed the number of participants lost to follow-up every 2 years. These data suggest censoring occurred randomly, independent of the event.

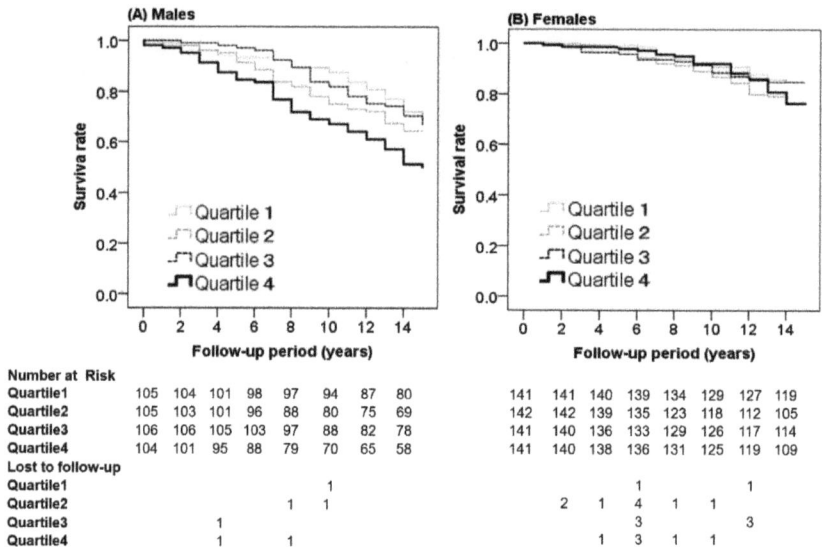

Figure 2. Kaplan–Meier survival curves showing the cumulative survival rate according to the FVC% predicted in males (**A**) and females (**B**).

Kaplan–Meier curves showing the cumulative survival rates according to Quartiles of % predicted value forced vital capacity (FVC% predicted). The cumulative survival rates were significantly lower in the lowest FVC% predicted group Quartile 4 in males (log-rank test, $p < 0.005$) but not in females (log-rank test, $p = 0.193$). The comparison between Quartile 4 and other groups: Q4 versus Q1; $p = 0.001$, Q4 versus Q2; $p = 0.040$, Q4 versus Q3; $p = 0.006$ in males. Q1; FVC% predicted ≥ 100.5 (male), ≥ 114.5 (female). Q2; FVC% predicted ≥ 89.2 to <100.5 (male), ≥ 100.9 to <114.5 (female). Q3; FVC% predicted ≥ 78.3 to <89.2 (male), ≥ 87.7 to <100.9 (female). Q4; FVC% predicted <78.3 (male), <87.7 (female). The number at risk shows the number of individuals at risk of experiencing an event for each group every 2 years. The lost to follow-up ratio shows the number of participants lost to follow-up for each group every 2 years.

Table 2 shows the association between the FVC% predicted divided into quartiles and mortality in males. Since the Kaplan–Meier survival curve of females divided into four groups by FVC% predicted could not show differences, we showed the data of males in the following analysis using quartile FVC% predicted. The highest FVC% predicted group (Q1) was set as a reference. Model 1 was a univariate model, and Model 2 was adjusted for multiple covariates. In males, lower FVC% predicted was inversely associated with higher mortality; the multivariate-adjusted HRs (95% CIs) was 2.12 (1.31 to 3.43) for the lowest FVC% predicted group Q4, which was significantly associated with higher mortality (p for trend = 0.010 in Model 3).

Table 2. Association between FVC% predicted divided into quartiles and mortality *.

	Males (420)				
	Q1 §	Q2 **	Q3 ††	Q4 ‡‡	p-trend
Number of cases	105	105	106	104	
Number of death	31	37	35	51	
Model 1 †	1.0 (ref.)	1.31 (0.81–2.11)	1.14 (0.70–1.85)	2.03 (1.30–3.18)	0.006
Model 2 ‡	1.0 (ref.)	1.48 (0.90–2.43)	1.18 (0.70–1.98)	2.12 (1.31–3.43)	0.010

FVC% predicted = % predicted value forced vital capacity; BMI = body mass index; hs-CRP = high sensitive C-reactive protein, ref = reference. * Hazard ratio (95% confidence interval). † Model 1: univariate model. ‡ Model 2: adjusted for age, medical history (pneumonia, bronchial asthma, cancer, stroke, myocardial infarction, diabetes, hypertension), smoking, alcohol consumption, depressive symptoms, cognitive function, educational level, marital status, leg extension power, BMI, albumin and hs-CRP. § Q1; FVC% predicted ≥100.5. ** Q2; FVC% predicted ≥89.2 to <100.5. †† Q3; FVC% predicted ≥78.3 to <89.2. ‡‡ Q4; FVC% predicted <78.3.

We then conducted sensitivity analyses for males. The results did not change after excluding cases who died in the first 3 years of follow-up (Supplementary Table S1).

Males were divided into four groups by leg power: The strongest Quartile 1 (w/kg): ≥15.8; Quartile 2: ≥13.1 to <15.8; Quartile 3: ≥10.8 to <13.1 and the weakest Quartile 4: <10.8. Table 3 shows the effect of muscle strength on the association between FVC% predicted and mortality. Model 1 showed that the HR (95% CI) of the lowest FVC% predicted group Q4 was 2.03 (1.30 to 3.18). In Model 2, the leg extension power was added to Model 1 as an explanatory variable, and the strongest leg power group Q1 was set as a reference. The HR of the lowest FVC% predicted group Q4 reduced to 1.78 (1.12 to 2.80) in Model 2 from 2.03 in Model 1. Leg power was significantly associated with mortality independently from FVC% predicted (p for trend = 0.025 in model 2). The weakest leg power group Q4 showed a HR of 1.67 (1.02 to 2.74), significantly associated with higher mortality.

Table 3. The effect of muscle strength on the association between FVC% predicted divided into quartiles and mortality *.

	Males (420)				
	Q1 ‖	Q2 **	Q3 ††	Q4 ‡‡	p-trend
Number of cases					
FVC% predicted	105	105	106	104	
Leg power	107	105	107	101	
Model 1 †					
FVC% predicted	1.0 (ref.)	1.31 (0.81–2.11)	1.14 (0.70–1.85)	2.03 (1.30–3.18)	0.006
Leg power	-	-	-	-	-
Model 2 ‡					
FVC% predicted	1.0 (ref.)	1.26 (0.78–2.03)	1.06 (0.65–1.72)	1.78 (1.12–2.80)	0.036
Leg power		1.43 (0.87–2.35)	1.79 (1.10–2.90)	1.67 (1.02–2.74)	0.025
Model 3 §					
FVC% predicted	1.0 (ref.)	1.48 (0.90–2.43)	1.18 (0.70–1.98)	2.12 (1.31–3.43)	0.010
Leg power		1.41 (0.84–2.38)	1.92 (1.15–3.23)	1.69 (0.96–2.98)	0.039

FVC% predicted = % predicted value forced vital capacity; BMI = body mass index; hs-CRP = high sensitive C-reactive protein, ref = reference. * Hazard ratio (95% confidence interval). † Model 1: univariate model. ‡ Model 2: Model 1+ leg extension power divided into quartiles. § Model 3: Model 2 adjusted for age, medical history (pneumonia, bronchial asthma, cancer, stroke, myocardial infarction, diabetes, hypertension), smoking, alcohol consumption, depressive symptoms, cognitive function, educational level, marital status, BMI, albumin and hs-CRP. ‖ Q1; FVC% predicted ≥100.5 & leg extension power ≥15.8, reference. ** Q2; FVC% predicted ≥89.2 to <100.5 & leg extension power ≥13.1 to <15.8. †† Q3; FVC% predicted ≥78.3 to <89.2 & leg extension power ≥10.8 to <13.1. ‡‡ Q4; FVC% predicted <78.3 & leg extension power <10.8.

To evaluate the relationship between the FVC% predicted, leg power, and mortality, we divided the subjects into a total of four groups by the clinical cut-off value of FVC% predicted (<80% group and ≥80% group) and by leg power (the strongest 25% group and the other groups), respectively (Table 4). The group with high FVC% predicted and strong leg power was set as a reference. Model 1 was a univariate model, and Model 2 was adjusted for multiple covariates. In Model 2, among low FVC% predicted males, the HRs were 2.69 (1.56 to 4.66) in the weak and 1.55 (0.58 to 4.15) in the strong leg power groups. The HRs showed similar trends in Models 1 and 2. The above findings suggest the potential unfavorable effects of weak leg power on the mortality of males among the low FVC% predicted subjects.

Table 4. The relationship between the leg power (2 groups), FVC% predicted (2 groups), and mortality *.

	Males (420)			
	FVC% predicted ≥80% strong leg power §	FVC% predicted ≥80% weak leg power **	FVC% predicted <80% strong leg power	FVC% predicted <80% weak leg power
Number of cases	91	205	16	108
Number of death	22	75	5	52
Model 1 [†]	1.0 (ref.)	1.63 (1.02–2.63)	1.38 (0.52–3.64)	2.44 (1.48–4.02)
Model 2 [‡]	1.0 (ref.)	1.69 (1.01–2.82)	1.55 (0.58–4.15)	2.69 (1.56–4.66)

FVC% predicted = % predicted value forced vital capacity; BMI = body mass index; hs-CRP = high sensitive C-reactive protein, ref = reference. * Hazard ratio (95% confidence interval). [†] Model 1: univariate model. [‡] Model 2: adjusted for age, medical history (pneumonia, bronchial asthma, cancer, stroke, myocardial infarction, diabetes, hypertension), smoking, alcohol consumption, depressive symptoms, cognitive function, educational level, marital status, BMI, albumin and hs-CRP. § Leg extension power ≥15.8 w/kg. ** Leg extension power <15.8 w/kg.

We then used the FVC% predicted 80% and divided the subjects into two groups. Supplementary Table S2 shows the association between the FVC% predicted (<80% group and ≥80% group) and mortality in males and females. The higher FVC% predicted ≥80% group was set as a reference. In both males and females, lower FVC% predicted was significantly associated with higher mortality. Males: HR 1.58 (1.11 to 2.24) and females: 1.87 (1.11 to 3.14) in Model 2.

Finally, the subjects were divided by gender and then into two groups by leg power (the strongest 25% group and the other groups). Supplementary Table S3 shows the effect of muscle strength on the association between FVC% predicted (<80% group and ≥80% group) and mortality. In females, Model 1 showed that the HR (95% Cl) of the low FVC% predicted group was 1.67 (1.05 to 2.64). In Model 2, the leg extension power was added to Model 1 as an explanatory variable, and the strong leg power group was set as a reference. The HRs of the low FVC% predicted groups essentially did not change, 1.67 (1.05 to 2.67) in Model 2 and 1.81 in (1.08 to 3.02) Model 3. Leg power was not associated with mortality. The weak leg power group showed a HR of 0.98 (0.63 to 1.52) in Model 2 and 1.05 (0.61 to 1.79) in Model 3. In males, the effect of muscle strength on the association between FVC% predicted and mortality showed a similar trend to Table 3, which was divided into four groups. Overall, the above findings suggest that weak leg power did not affect the mortality of females among the low FVC% predicted group.

4. Discussion

Lower FVC% predicted was associated with a higher risk of all-cause mortality in community-dwelling older males without respiratory symptoms. FVC% predicted under 80% was a risk factor for all-cause mortality in females. Weak leg power may have the potential to unfavorably affect the association in males with low FVC% predicted but not in females.

This study showed that weak leg power was associated with high mortality in community-dwelling older males. Previous studies showed an association between weak extremity muscle power, including leg power and high mortality [11–16]. We could not find such an association in females. However, a previous study could not show an association in older Japanese females [13]. This may reflect the differences in ethnicity or lifestyles between Japanese/east Asians and people in other countries.

Previous studies showing an association between low FVC and high mortality did not mention factors that can affect the risk [1–6,9,10]. This study showed a dose-response relationship between higher FVC% predicted and lower male mortality. Furthermore, when leg power was put into the model as an explanatory variable, the variable was independently associated with mortality and reduced the HR of the low FVC% predicted. This suggests that weak leg power may predict the high mortality of low FVC% predicted. Indeed, analysis of the subjects divided into four groups by the FVC% predicted (two groups) and leg power (two groups) showed a trend of high mortality risk in the weak leg power group than in the strong leg power group among low FVC% predicted males. However, the number of males with low FVC% predicted and strong leg power was insufficient.

The cause of death from low FVC in people without respiratory symptoms is unclear [9]. For extremity muscles, weak leg power was associated with high-pneumonia mortality in older males, but the mechanisms were unclear [31]. Respiratory function and extremity muscle power moderately correlate with respiratory muscle strength [17–20]. The respiratory muscle strength has a clear relationship with pneumonia. Strong respiratory muscles generate effective coughing, clear the airways, and prevent pneumonia [18,21,32,33]. Indeed, respiratory muscle weakness was a risk factor for the onset of and possibly death by pneumonia in older people [21]. Muscle weakness is related to inflammation, including pneumonia [34–37]. Thus, the association between weak extremity muscle power and pneumonia might be mediated through respiratory muscle weakness. Likewise, low FVC% predicted might be associated with pneumonia through respiratory muscle weakness. From the point of view of muscle weakness, asymptomatic neuromuscular diseases can cause death. Furthermore, considering respiratory muscle weakness, diaphragmatic dysfunction, such as diaphragmatic nerve paralysis, can also cause death.

Females showed an association between low FVC% predicted under 80% and high mortality, and leg power did not affect this association. Thus, in older Japanese females, associations between respiratory muscle strength, leg power, and lung function might be weak, or other unknown factors might be involved.

A previous study suggested that FVC was not associated with mortality in older people without respiratory symptoms [10]. This discrepancy is possibly due to their 8-year follow-up. In contrast, it was 15 years in our study, in which the analysis was of FVC instead of FVC% predicted, or did not include dyspnea as a respiratory symptom.

Forced expiratory volume in 1 second (FEV1.0) is another major indicator of respiratory functions with its well-known association with mortality, and its value is greatly worsened by smoking [1,5]. Since the effects of smoking on FEV1.0 were extremely great [1,3,5], we had difficulties analyzing the effects of muscle power on the association between FEV1.0 and mortality.

We calculated the sample size of our main result; the lower FVC% predicted males exhibited higher mortality risks. The power for males' Q1 and Q4 hazard ratios was 0.89, which suggests a sufficient sample size for the analysis.

This study has some limitations. First, this study could not examine the association between FVC% predicted and cause-specific mortality. Therefore, other data sets will be required to identify the association. Second, the ethnicity was limited to Japanese. Third, we could not identify factors that affect the high mortality in females with low FVC% predicted. Fourth, we could not completely exclude potential interstitial lung disease patients since they can present asymptomatic and with normal pulmonary function tests.

The present study suggests that low FVC% predicted is associated with an increased risk of all-cause mortality in community-dwelling older people without respiratory symptoms. In addition, this study suggests that weak leg power predicts a high risk of death due to the low FVC% predicted in older males. Hence, we may highlight the increased risk to such males in various situations, such as in clinical settings and medical examinations.

Supplementary Materials: The following supporting information can be downloaded at: https://www.mdpi.com/article/10.3390/jcm11185264/s1, Table S1: Association between FVC% predicted and mortality (Exclusion of deaths occurring in the first 3 years of follow-up); Table S2: Association between FVC% predicted (2 groups <80% and ≥80%) and mortality; Table S3: The effect of muscle strength (two groups) * on the association between FVC% predicted (two groups <80% and ≥80%) and mortality.

Author Contributions: M.M.: Methodology, formal analysis, and writing; T.O.: Conceptualization, investigation, funding acquisition, and writing; Y.S.: Methodology, formal analysis, and writing; S.M.: Data curation, project administration, and resources; I.T.: Data curation, investigation, project administration, resources, supervision, and writing; S.-I.I.: Conceptualization, funding acquisition, and supervision. All authors have read and agreed to the published version of the manuscript.

Funding: This work was supported by a Grant-In-Aid for Scientific Research from the Ministry of Education, Science and Culture of the Japanese Government (18K08133, 22H02964), Japan Agency for Medical Research and Development (17dk0110024), and The General Insurance Association of Japan to Tatsuma Okazaki. Japan Agency for Medical Research and Development (20dk0310101h0002) to Tatsuma Okazaki. and Shin-Ichi Izumi.

Institutional Review Board Statement: The study was conducted according to the guidelines of the Declaration of Helsinki and approved by the Ethics Committee of Tohoku University Graduate School of Medicine (approval number: 2002040).

Informed Consent Statement: Informed consent was obtained from all subjects involved in the study.

Data Availability Statement: Data are available upon reasonable request.

Acknowledgments: The authors thank Brent Bell for reading the manuscript.

Conflicts of Interest: The authors declare no conflict of interest.

References

1. Honda, Y.; Watanabe, T.; Shibata, Y.; Otaki, Y.; Kadowaki, S.; Narumi, T.; Takahashi, T.; Kinoshita, D.; Yokoyama, M.; Nishiyama, S.; et al. Impact of restrictive lung disorder on cardiovascular mortality in a general population: The Yamagata (Takahata) study. *Int. J. Cardiol.* **2017**, *241*, 395–400. [CrossRef]
2. Scarlata, S.; Pedone, C.; Fimognari, F.L.; Bellia, V.; Forastiere, F.; Incalzi, R.A. Restrictive pulmonary dysfunction at spirometry and mortality in the elderly. *Respir. Med.* **2008**, *102*, 1349–1354. [CrossRef] [PubMed]
3. Magnussen, C.; Ojeda, F.M.; Rzayeva, N.; Zeller, T.; Sinning, C.R.; Pfeiffer, N.; Beutel, M.; Blettner, M.; Lackner, K.J.; Blankenberg, S.; et al. FEV1 and FVC predict all-cause mortality independent of cardiac function—Results from the population-based Gutenberg Health Study. *Int. J. Cardiol.* **2017**, *234*, 64–68. [CrossRef]
4. Breet, Y.; Schutte, A.E.; Huisman, H.W.; Eloff, F.C.; Du Plessis, J.L.; Kruger, A.; Van Rooyen, J.M. Lung function, inflammation and cardiovascular mortality in Africans. *Eur. J. Clin. Invest.* **2016**, *46*, 901–910. [CrossRef] [PubMed]
5. Mannino, D.M.; Buist, A.S.; Petty, T.L.; Enright, P.L.; Redd, S.C. Lung function and mortality in the United States: Data from the First National Health and Nutrition Examination Survey follow up study. *Thorax* **2003**, *58*, 388–393. [CrossRef] [PubMed]
6. Vaz Fragoso, C.A.; Van Ness, P.H.; Murphy, T.E.; McAvay, G.J. Spirometric impairments, cardiovascular outcomes, and noncardiovascular death in older persons. *Respir. Med.* **2018**, *137*, 40–47. [CrossRef]
7. Putman, R.K.; Hatabu, H.; Araki, T.; Gudmundsson, G.; Gao, W.; Nishino, M.; Okajima, Y.; Dupuis, J.; Latourelle, J.C.; Cho, M.H.; et al. Association Between Interstitial Lung Abnormalities and All-Cause Mortality. *JAMA* **2016**, *315*, 672–681. [CrossRef]
8. Wise, J. Interstitial lung abnormalities are linked to increased risk of death. *BMJ* **2016**, *352*, i971. [CrossRef]
9. Burney, P.G.; Hooper, R. Forced vital capacity, airway obstruction and survival in a general population sample from the USA. *Thorax* **2011**, *66*, 49–54. [CrossRef]
10. Weinmayr, G.; Schulz, H.; Klenk, J.; Denkinger, M.; Duran-Tauleria, E.; Koenig, W.; Dallmeier, D.; Rothenbacher, D.; Acti, F.E.S.G. Association of lung function with overall mortality is independent of inflammatory, cardiac, and functional biomarkers in older adults: The ActiFE-study. *Sci. Rep.* **2020**, *10*, 11862. [CrossRef] [PubMed]
11. Laukkanen, P.; Heikkinen, E.; Kauppinen, M. Muscle strength and mobility as predictors of survival in 75–84-year-old people. *Age Ageing* **1995**, *24*, 468–473. [CrossRef] [PubMed]
12. Metter, E.J.; Talbot, L.A.; Schrager, M.; Conwit, R. Skeletal muscle strength as a predictor of all-cause mortality in healthy men. *J. Gerontol. A Biol. Sci. Med. Sci.* **2002**, *57*, B359–B365. [CrossRef]
13. Takata, Y.; Shimada, M.; Ansai, T.; Yoshitake, Y.; Nishimuta, M.; Nakagawa, N.; Ohashi, M.; Yoshihara, A.; Miyazaki, H. Physical performance and 10-year mortality in a 70-year-old community-dwelling population. *Aging Clin. Exp. Res.* **2012**, *24*, 257–264. [CrossRef] [PubMed]
14. Celis-Morales, C.A.; Welsh, P.; Lyall, D.M.; Steell, L.; Petermann, F.; Anderson, J.; Iliodromiti, S.; Sillars, A.; Graham, N.; Mackay, D.F.; et al. Associations of grip strength with cardiovascular, respiratory, and cancer outcomes and all cause mortality: Prospective cohort study of half a million UK Biobank participants. *BMJ* **2018**, *361*, k1651. [CrossRef] [PubMed]

15. Newman, A.B.; Kupelian, V.; Visser, M.; Simonsick, E.M.; Goodpaster, B.H.; Kritchevsky, S.B.; Tylavsky, F.A.; Rubin, S.M.; Harris, T.B. Strength, but not muscle mass, is associated with mortality in the health, aging and body composition study cohort. *J. Gerontol. A Biol. Sci. Med. Sci.* **2006**, *61*, 72–77. [CrossRef] [PubMed]
16. Gale, C.R.; Martyn, C.N.; Cooper, C.; Sayer, A.A. Grip strength, body composition, and mortality. *Int. J. Epidemiol.* **2007**, *36*, 228–235. [CrossRef]
17. Enright, P.L.; Kronmal, R.A.; Manolio, T.A.; Schenker, M.B.; Hyatt, R.E. Respiratory muscle strength in the elderly. Correlates and reference values. Cardiovascular Health Study Research Group. *Am. J. Respir. Crit. Care Med.* **1994**, *149*, 430–438. [CrossRef] [PubMed]
18. Okazaki, T.; Ebihara, S.; Mori, T.; Izumi, S.; Ebihara, T. Association between sarcopenia and pneumonia in older people. *Geriatr. Gerontol. Int.* **2020**, *20*, 7–13. [CrossRef] [PubMed]
19. Shin, H.I.; Kim, D.K.; Seo, K.M.; Kang, S.H.; Lee, S.Y.; Son, S. Relation Between Respiratory Muscle Strength and Skeletal Muscle Mass and Hand Grip Strength in the Healthy Elderly. *Ann. Rehabil. Med.* **2017**, *41*, 686–692. [CrossRef] [PubMed]
20. Buchman, A.S.; Boyle, P.A.; Wilson, R.S.; Gu, L.; Bienias, J.L.; Bennett, D.A. Pulmonary function, muscle strength and mortality in old age. *Mech. Ageing Dev.* **2008**, *129*, 625–631. [CrossRef]
21. Okazaki, T.; Suzukamo, Y.; Miyatake, M.; Komatsu, R.; Yaekashiwa, M.; Nihei, M.; Izumi, S.; Ebihara, T. Respiratory Muscle Weakness as a Risk Factor for Pneumonia in Older People. *Gerontology* **2021**, *67*, 581–590. [CrossRef] [PubMed]
22. Hozawa, A.; Ohmori, K.; Kuriyama, S.; Shimazu, T.; Niu, K.; Watando, A.; Ebihara, S.; Matsui, T.; Ichiki, M.; Nagatomi, R.; et al. C-reactive protein and peripheral artery disease among Japanese elderly: The Tsurugaya Project. *Hypertens. Res.* **2004**, *27*, 955–961. [CrossRef]
23. Kuriyama, S.; Hozawa, A.; Ohmori, K.; Shimazu, T.; Matsui, T.; Ebihara, S.; Awata, S.; Nagatomi, R.; Arai, H.; Tsuji, I. Green tea consumption and cognitive function: A cross-sectional study from the Tsurugaya Project 1. *Am. J. Clin. Nutr.* **2006**, *83*, 355–361. [CrossRef] [PubMed]
24. Ebihara, S.; Niu, K.; Ebihara, T.; Kuriyama, S.; Hozawa, A.; Ohmori-Matsuda, K.; Nakaya, N.; Nagatomi, R.; Arai, H.; Kohzuki, M.; et al. Impact of blunted perception of dyspnea on medical care use and expenditure, and mortality in elderly people. *Front. Physiol.* **2012**, *3*, 238. [CrossRef] [PubMed]
25. Kanezaki, M.; Terada, K.; Ebihara, S. Effect of Olfactory Stimulation by L-Menthol on Laboratory-Induced Dyspnea in COPD. *Chest* **2020**, *157*, 1455–1465. [CrossRef] [PubMed]
26. Kubota, M.; Kobayashi, H.; Quanjer, P.H.; Omori, H.; Tatsumi, K.; Kanazawa, M.; Clinical Pulmonary Functions Committee of the Japanese Respiratory Society. Reference values for spirometry, including vital capacity, in Japanese adults calculated with the LMS method and compared with previous values. *Respir. Investig.* **2014**, *52*, 242–250. [CrossRef] [PubMed]
27. Standardization of Spirometry, 1994 Update. American Thoracic Society. *Am. J. Respir. Crit. Care Med.* **1995**, *152*, 1107–1136. [CrossRef]
28. Yang, G.; Niu, K.; Fujita, K.; Hozawa, A.; Ohmori-Matsuda, K.; Kuriyama, S.; Nakaya, N.; Ebihara, S.; Okazaki, T.; Guo, H.; et al. Impact of physical activity and performance on medical care costs among the Japanese elderly. *Geriatr. Gerontol. Int.* **2011**, *11*, 157–165. [CrossRef]
29. Kuriyama, S.; Koizumi, Y.; Matsuda-Ohmori, K.; Seki, T.; Shimazu, T.; Hozawa, A.; Awata, S.; Tsuji, I. Obesity and depressive symptoms in elderly Japanese: The Tsurugaya Project. *J. Psychosom. Res.* **2006**, *60*, 229–235. [CrossRef]
30. Folstein, M.F.; Folstein, S.E.; McHugh, P.R. "Mini-mental state". A practical method for grading the cognitive state of patients for the clinician. *J. Psychiatr. Res.* **1975**, *12*, 189–198. [CrossRef]
31. Takata, Y.; Ansai, T.; Akifusa, S.; Soh, I.; Yoshitake, Y.; Kimura, Y.; Sonoki, K.; Fujisawa, K.; Awano, S.; Kagiyama, S.; et al. Physical fitness and 4-year mortality in an 80-year-old population. *J. Gerontol. A Biol. Sci. Med. Sci.* **2007**, *62*, 851–858. [CrossRef] [PubMed]
32. American Thoracic Society/European Respiratory Society. ATS/ERS Statement on respiratory muscle testing. *Am. J. Respir. Crit. Care Med.* **2002**, *166*, 518–624. [CrossRef]
33. Ebihara, S.; Sekiya, H.; Miyagi, M.; Ebihara, T.; Okazaki, T. Dysphagia, dystussia, and aspiration pneumonia in elderly people. *J. Thorac. Dis.* **2016**, *8*, 632–639. [CrossRef] [PubMed]
34. Komatsu, R.; Okazaki, T.; Ebihara, S.; Kobayashi, M.; Tsukita, Y.; Nihei, M.; Sugiura, H.; Niu, K.; Ebihara, T.; Ichinose, M. Aspiration pneumonia induces muscle atrophy in the respiratory, skeletal, and swallowing systems. *J. Cachexia Sarcopenia Muscle* **2018**, *9*, 643–653. [CrossRef]
35. Okazaki, T.; Liang, F.; Li, T.; Lemaire, C.; Danialou, G.; Shoelson, S.E.; Petrof, B.J. Muscle-specific inhibition of the classical nuclear factor-kappaB pathway is protective against diaphragmatic weakness in murine endotoxemia. *Crit. Care Med.* **2014**, *42*, e501–e509. [CrossRef]
36. Supinski, G.S.; Morris, P.E.; Dhar, S.; Callahan, L.A. Diaphragm Dysfunction in Critical Illness. *Chest* **2018**, *153*, 1040–1051. [CrossRef]
37. Petrof, B.J. Diaphragm Weakness in the Critically Ill: Basic Mechanisms Reveal Therapeutic Opportunities. *Chest* **2018**, *154*, 1395–1403. [CrossRef] [PubMed]

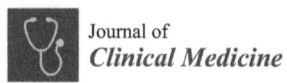

Review

Are Oropharyngeal Dysphagia Screening Tests Effective in Preventing Pneumonia?

Ikuko Okuni and Satoru Ebihara *

Department of Rehabilitation Medicine, Toho University Graduate School of Medicine, Tokyo 143-8541, Japan; pon1990@med.toho-u.ac.jp
* Correspondence: satoru.ebihara@med.toho-u.ac.jp; Tel.: +81-3-3762-4151

Abstract: Oropharyngeal dysphagia, a clinical condition that indicates difficulty in moving food and liquid from the oral cavity to the esophagus, has a markedly high prevalence in the elderly. The number of elderly people with oropharyngeal dysphagia is expected to increase due to the aging of the world's population. Understanding the current situation of dysphagia screening is crucial when considering future countermeasures. We report findings from a literature review including citations on current objective dysphagia screening tests: the Water Swallowing Test, Mann Assessment of Swallowing Ability, and the Gugging Swallowing Screen. Pneumonia can be predicted using the results of the screening tests discussed in this review, and the response after the screening tests is important for prevention. In addition, although interdisciplinary team approaches prevent and reduce aspiration, optimal treatment is a challenging. Intervention studies with multiple factors focusing on the elderly are needed.

Keywords: dysphagia; aspiration; screening; water swallowing test; Mann Assessment of Swallowing Ability; Gugging Swallowing Screen

1. Introduction

Oropharyngeal dysphagia is a clinical condition characterized by difficulties in moving food and liquid from the oral cavity to the esophagus. The prevalence of oropharyngeal dysphagia is markedly high; 16% of elderly individuals aged 70–79 years who live independently suffer from oropharyngeal dysphagia, increasing to 33% in those aged 80 years or older. Moreover, 51% of the elderly aged 65 years or older living in institutions suffer from dysphagia [1]. Thus, oropharyngeal dysphagia has a markedly high prevalence. Furthermore, the prevalence of many diseases that can cause oropharyngeal dysphagia increases with age. Thus, it has been suggested that age-related changes contribute to oropharyngeal dysphagia. The international trend of aging shows that the proportion of people aged 65 years and older in the total population (population aging rate) has risen from 5.1% in 1950 to 8.3% in 2015, and it is expected to rise to 17.8% by 2060. Population aging will likely progress rapidly in the next half of this century [2]. As such, the number of elderly people with oropharyngeal dysphagia is expected to increase worldwide.

Oropharyngeal dysphagia can cause loss of appetite, malnutrition, and poor physical function; it can ultimately lead to life-threatening situations such as aspiration pneumonia and asphyxiation accidents. Therefore, understanding the current oropharyngeal dysphagia situation is crucial, especially when considering countermeasures for the future. In recent years, the recommendation to restart oral intake early to maintain swallowing function and shorten the treatment period, if possible, even in patients with acute aspiration pneumonia, has been advocated [3]. Swallowing function can be evaluated using a variety of methods, including interviews, medical examinations, screenings, and evaluative tests using specialized equipment. Through conversations with patients and their families, interviews systematically collect the information necessary for diagnosis, match this information with medical knowledge, and draw inferences to formulate and direct diagnosis; thus, interviews are an important first step in the care process. Specifically, interviews are essential for obtaining comprehensive medical histories and identifying symptoms suspected to cause oropharyngeal dysphagia, as well as systemic symptoms, such as nutritional and respiratory status. Symptoms associated with oropharyngeal dysphagia can be systematically identified using designated questionnaires. The accuracy of some of these questionnaires, including the Seirei Dysphagia Screening Questionnaire and the Eating Assessment Tool-10 (EAT-10), has been validated for dysphagia screening. Subjective screening questionnaires in the elderly may reduce the prevalence of oropharyngeal dysphagia, due to factors such as unawareness of swallowing problems, swallowing difficulties perceived as natural consequences of aging, and the presence of silent aspiration. Therefore, the use of subjective dysphagia screening in combination with objective dysphagia screening increases the prevalence of oropharyngeal dysphagia [4]. Ideally, such screening should yield a positive result for all individuals with oropharyngeal dysphagia (sensitivity) and a negative result for all individuals without it (specificity), which can be carried out without the use of special equipment. An ideal screening instrument is highly needed in medical institutions, long-term care facilities, nursing facilities, and visiting care settings where equipment is not available. Moreover, with an ideal screening test, unnecessary referrals and tests may be reduced. Furthermore, dysphagia screening should be able to prevent aspiration pneumonia. Here, we conducted a literature review on non-instrumental, objective dysphagia screening tests and outlined their effectiveness in preventing pneumonia.

2. Literature Search on Dysphagia Screening

In order to understand the current status of non-instrumental objective screening tests in recent years, we conducted a literature search to identify screening tests that have been suggested to be effective and have been used in multiple institutions (Figure 1).

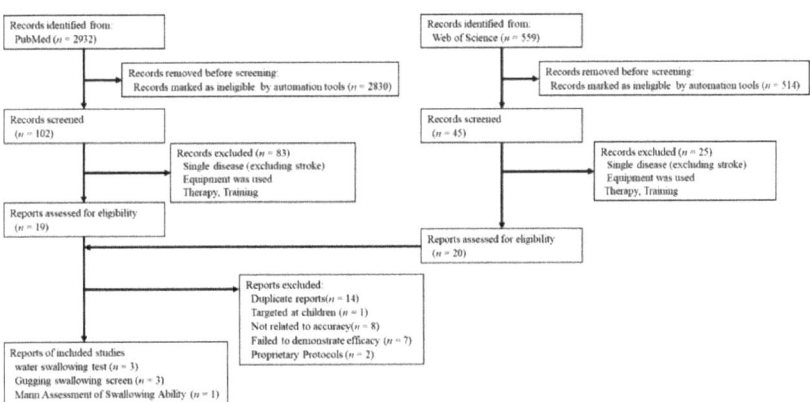

Figure 1. Study selection flowchart.

In the first step, we defined the four elements of the clinical question as follows: population: elderly people with suspected dysphagia; intervention: non-instrumental screening tests; comparison: instrumental tests (fiberoptic endoscopic swallow study, videofluoroscopic swallow study); and outcome: effectiveness of the diagnosis of aspiration. This was then followed by a search for articles using a structural formula that combines the words "dysphagia", "aspiration", and "screening" screening in PubMed-yielded 2932 articles. We then narrowed down the article search to meta-analyses, randomized controlled trials, and systematic reviews published within the last 10 years (from January 2011 to July 2021), which yielded 102 articles. We tried to limit the number of papers to those that studied the elderly, but there were too few, so we instead excluded papers on single diseases only, excluding stroke. Furthermore, we excluded studies that used equipment such as fiberoptic endoscopic swallow studies and videofluoroscopic swallow studies, and those related to oral care, treatment, and training. Subsequently, 19 suitable articles were identified. A similar search and exclusion process using the Web of Science database resulted in 20 papers. After reading the articles, we excluded duplicates (n = 14), an article examining children (n = 1), those not related to the accuracy of screening tests (n = 8), and systematic reviews that failed to indicate the effectiveness of screening tests (n = 7). We additionally excluded a randomized controlled trial using the DREP screening (DREPs) [5], which is a protocol used in Brazil, and a randomized controlled trial using an original semi-solid swallowing test [6], as these are conducted in few facilities. We found three systematic reviews related to the water swallowing test [7–9], indicating that it is the most common screening test. Systematic reviews of effective swallowing screening for acute stroke [10] and swallowing screening in nursing homes [11] showed that the Gugging Swallowing Screen is a highly reliable tool with high sensitivity. In addition, a 2020 systematic review of the Gugging Swallowing Screen showed similar results [12], indicating that the Gugging Swallowing Screen is an effective screening test that can be used in different facilities. Perren et al. conducted a systematic review to evaluate post-extubation dysphagia in critically ill patients [13]. Despite the lack of available data on dysphagia screening in intensive care settings, they stated that the Mann Assessment of Swallowing Ability might serve as a reliable validated tool for diagnosing dysphagia in stroke patients. Based on these reports, we examined three dysphagia screening tests: the Water Swallowing Test, Mann Assessment of Swallowing Ability, and Gugging Swallowing Screen. The original articles discussed in the adopted reviews, including citations, are presented in Table 1. However, the articles were limited to those with a sample size of at least 40, and we divided the protocols for the Water Swallowing Test into three types (single sips, consecutive sips, and progressive amounts). Each of the three articles was excerpted in chronological order from the most recent to the oldest.

Table 1. Dysphagia screening methods (sensitivity and specificity).

Study (Year)	Patients Included (Etiology)	Swallowing Assessment Method	Inspector	Reference Test	Outcome	Sensitivity	Specificity
Wakasugi et al. [14]. (2008)	107 (MD)	Water Swallowing Test Single sips 3 mL, Total amount 3 mL	NR	VFSS, FEES	Aspiration	69	97
Momosaki et al. [15]. (2013)	110 (CVA)	Single sips 4 mL, Total amount ≤12	SLP	FEES	Aspiration	93	79
McCullough et al. [16]. (2005)	165 (CVA)	Single sips 5 mL, Total amount ≤10	Doctor	VFSS	Aspiration	44	94
		Single sips 10 mL, Total amount ≤20	Doctor	VFSS	Aspiration	37	96
Suiter et al. [17]. (2008)	3000 (MD)	Consecutive sips 90 mL	Doctor	FEES	Aspiration	97	49
Zhou et al. [18]. (2011)	107 (CVA)	Consecutive sips 90 mL	Doctor	VFSS	Aspiration	87	42
Patterson et al. [19]. (2011)	126 (HNC)	Consecutive sips 100 mL	NR	FEES	Aspiration	80	77
Hey et al. [20]. (2013)	80 (HNC)	Progressive amounts 2, 5, 10, 20 mL Total amount ≤51 mL	SLP	FEES	Aspiration	100	61
Somasundaram et al. [21]. (2014)	67 (CVA)	Progressive amounts 5, 10, 20 mL Total amount ≤50 mL	SLP	VFSS	Aspiration	70	81
Hassan et al. [22]. (2014)	74 (MD)	Progressive amounts 5, 20, 50 mL Total amount ≤75 mL	NR	FEES	Aspiration	74	70
Mann et al. [23]. (2000)	128 (CVA)	MASA	SLP	VFSS	Swallowing disorder	73	89

Table 1. Cont.

Study (Year)	Patients Included (Etiology)	Swallowing Assessment Method	Inspector	Reference Test	Outcome	Sensitivity	Specificity
González-Fernández et al. [24]. (2011)	133 (MD)	MASA	SLP	VFSS	Aspiration	39.6	59
Antonios et al. [25]. (2010)	150 (CVA)	Modified MASA	Doctor	MASA	Swallowing disorder	87~92	84.2~86.3
Trapl et al. [26]. (2007)	50 (CVA)	GUSS	SLP Nurse	FEES	Aspiration	100	50~69
Warnecke et al. [27]. (2017)	100 (CVA)	GUSS	SLP	FEES	Aspiration	96.5	55.8
Said Bassiouny et al. [28]. (2017)	40 (CVA)	GUSS	SLP	FEES	Aspiration	93.8	96.1

CVA: cerebrovascular accident, HNC: head and neck cancer, MD: mixed-disease. SLP: speech-language pathologist, NR: not reported. VFSS: videofluoroscopic swallow study, FEES: fiberoptic endoscopic swallow study; MASA: Mann Assessment of Swallowing Ability, GUSS: Gugging Swallowing Screen. All solids in the GUSS were dry bread.

We reviewed the methodological quality of each included study, using criteria from the Quality Assessment of Studies of Diagnostic Accuracy (QUADAS-2) tool, as recommended by Cochrane (www.quadas.org; accessed on 12 December 2021). Results of the methodological quality assessment for each of the 15 included studies are shown in Table 2. We considered three studies to be at low risk across all four risk-of-bias domains: patient selection, index test, reference standard, and flow and timing (McCullough et al. [16], Trapl et al. [26], and Warnecke et al. [27]). Three studies were at low risk of bias for three domains (Hey et al. [20], Mann et al. [23], and Antonios et al. [25]). A major concern for risk of bias across the other included studies was that they had not enrolled consecutive patients or were unknown. In addition, some studies adopted a convenience sampling method. Finally, there were a number of high-risk studies due to the fact that they were carried out by people who knew the respective results of the index test and the reference standard. It was also unclear in eight studies whether there was an appropriate time interval between the index test and the reference standard. There were no applicability concerns for 15 studies across the three applicability domains: patient selection, index test, and reference standard.

Table 2. Assessment of the quality of the included studies.

Study (Year)	Risk of Bias				Applicability Concerns		
	Patient Selection	Index Test	Reference Standard	Flow and Timing	Patient Selection	Index Test	Reference Standard
Wakasugi et al. [14]. (2008)	-	-	?	?	+	+	+
Momosaki et al. [15]. (2013)	-	+	?	+	+	+	+
McCullough et al. [16]. (2005)	+	+	+	+	+	+	+
Suiter et al. [17]. (2008)	?	-	+	-	+	+	+
Zhou et al. [18]. (2011)	?	-	-	?	+	+	+
Patterson et al. [19]. (2011)	?	+	-	?	+	+	+
Hey et al. [20]. (2013)	?	+	+	+	+	+	+
Somasundaram et al. [21]. (2014)	+	+	?	?	+	+	+
Hassan et al. [22]. (2014)	?	+	-	?	+	+	+
Mann et al. [23]. (2000)	+	+	+	?	+	+	+
Gonzá-lez-Fernández et al. [24]. (2011)	+	-	+	?	+	+	+
Antonios et al. [25]. (2010)	+	-	+	+	+	+	+
Trapl et al. [26]. (2007)	+	+	+	+	+	+	+
Warnecke et al. [27]. (2017)	+	+	+	+	+	+	+
Said Bas-siouny et al. [28]. (2017)	?	+	+	?	+	+	+

(+): Low Risk, (-): High Risk, (?): Unclear Risk. The risk of bias and applicability were assessed according to QUADAS-2 (www.quadas.org, accessed on 12 December 2021).

3. Water Swallowing Test

The amount of water used in the Water Swallowing Test (WST) varies, with 3–20 mL for single swallowing, 90–100 mL for continuous swallowing, and 2–50 mL for a titration method, which increases the amount of water in stages, each exhibiting varying levels of diagnostic accuracy (Table 1). Among these stages, the test has the most suitable characteristics for excluding aspiration when a certain amount of water (e.g., 90 mL), is continuously ingested. In addition, the WST, with a single ingestion of a small volume, was superior for correctly classifying aspirating patients. Therefore, it may be possible to increase the sensitivity and specificity within a screening session of the same patient by performing both continuous drinking of a certain amount and single drinking of a small amount in stages [7]. However, there are currently no articles on the WST that support a high sensitivity and high specificity, and continuous swallowing of 90 mL of water is not recommended for patients who have begun to show signs of dysphagia or require a tracheostomy tube to secure the airway [20,29].

A recent prospective study of 102 patients aged 75 years or older (mean age 84.5 years) who were admitted to a geriatric ward reported a sensitivity of 76.6% and specificity of 65% (examiner: physician) for continuous swallowing of 90 mL of water [30]. In a cross-sectional study of 94 community-dwelling older people (aged 65 years and over) living independently, there was no significant difference in maximum tongue pressure between the sarcopenic (47.0 kPa) and non-sarcopenic (48.6 kPa) groups, but the time taken to drink 100 mL of water was significantly longer in the sarcopenic group (12.43 s) than in the non-sarcopenic group (5.66 s). This finding suggests that sarcopenic patients have a reduced ability to swallow [31]. The cut-off value for tongue pressure in the diagnostic criteria for sarcopenic dysphagia is less than 20 kPa [32]. This delay may be an early predictor of dysphagia before clinical problems become apparent.

3.1. Research Results on WST and Pneumonia

Most studies evaluating the effectiveness of the WST and pneumonia prevention have been conducted in patients with a single disease. Miki et al. conducted a symptom questionnaire, the Repetitive Saliva Swallowing Test (RSST), and the WST for dysphagia screening using a single 30 mL intake protocol in 85 postoperative patients with stomach cancer [33]. The results showed that postoperative pneumonia was not observed in patients who tested positive in the screening tests. Furthermore, the authors reported that intervention by the rehabilitation department to which the positive patients were referred was important in reducing the incidence of pneumonia. Three patients who developed postoperative pneumonia tested negative in the screening tests, and the cause of pneumonia was thought to be an aspiration in all cases. These results suggest that the screening tests used in this study did not sufficiently identify patients at high risk for aspiration pneumonia.

Ebersole et al. examined the incidence of hospital-acquired aspiration pneumonia (HAAP) in 12,392 hospitalized cancer patients who did or did not participate in nursing-initiated dysphagia screenings [34]. The incidence of HAAP per 1000 discharged patients who underwent dysphagia screening by the WST (continuous swallowing of 90 mL of water) was 8.78, and that per 1000 discharged patients who did not undergo dysphagia screening was 7.36. The study reported that dysphagia screening had no apparent effect on the incidence of HAAP. However, patients at high risk of oropharyngeal dysphagia, such as those with a history of head and neck cancer, were excluded from the screening process in this study; instead, they underwent more comprehensive instrumental swallowing evaluations. In addition, 30% of HAAP patients associated with difficulty in swallowing were fasting prior to aspiration, highlighting the difficulty of preventing HAAP in this population. Discontinuing an oral diet is not equivalent to eliminating the risk of HAAP. The authors stated that aspiration of secretions, microaspiration of oropharyngeal bacteria, and reflux associated with tube feeding were the causes of HAAP risk, regardless of dietary status.

Oguchi et al. conducted a retrospective study of 97 post-extubation patients undergoing cardiovascular surgery [35]. The endpoints were consciousness level (Glasgow Coma Scale), RSST, WST (3 mL in single intake), speech intelligibility score, and risk of dysphagia in the cardiac surgery score (RODICS) [36]. They reported that WST was the strongest predictive factor of postoperative pneumonia compared to other evaluations and that the incidence of pneumonia increased approximately three-fold when aspiration was suspected by the WST. However, 57.14% of patients who did not start oral intake, according to the results of the WST, were subsequently diagnosed with pneumonia. The authors stated that it is important to analyze the causal mechanism and consider measures to prevent pneumonia, such as improvement in wakefulness, swallowing function training, assistance with phlegm expulsion, airway suction, postural drainage, and oral care.

3.2. Combining the WST with Other Screening Tests

Surprisingly, there are few articles on the WST and pneumonia prevention. As the WST evaluates airway response and voice changes, it may overlook silent aspiration, which is caused by the absence of a cough reflex or throat ringing even when a substance is absorbed in the subglottis. To compensate for this oversight, pulse oximetry, cervical auscultation, and cough tests were used in a combined evaluation. Pulse oximetry, which measures oxyhemoglobin saturation in peripheral capillaries, is used to detect a decrease in saturation that suggests aspiration during swallowing. However, the diagnostic accuracy of pulse oximetry in predicting aspiration is controversial, and current evidence does not support its use [37].

Cervical auscultation determines dysphagia, mainly in the pharyngeal phase, by listening to swallowing and breathing sounds using a stethoscope placed on the neck. Although it has long been used as a non-invasive and common screening method, it lacks sufficient objectivity and reliability among available evaluators because of the limitations of the human auditory system and the fact that the stethoscope is designed and tuned for a specific purpose, such as observing heart or lung sounds [38]. However, a device called high-resolution cervical auscultation (HRCA) has been developed, which is expected to be applied clinically as a non-invasive screening method and as a biofeedback method during treatment [39].

We did not find any studies evaluating the effectiveness of the WST in combination with pulse oximetry or cervical auscultation for preventing pneumonia, but one study investigated the association between the combined WST and cough test, and the onset of pneumonia, which is shown below. Nakamori et al. investigated the association between the RSST, the WST (3 mL in single intake), and a cough test with the onset of pneumonia in acute stroke patients [40]. Each test was performed on 226 patients upon admission; the patients were then monitored for 30 days. Of these, 17 patients developed pneumonia during the observation period, and the sensitivity and specificity of the WST were 29.4% and 95.2%, respectively. Other screening tests alone did not adequately predict the risk of aspiration pneumonia. However, combining these three tests increased the sensitivity and specificity to 88.2% and 83.7%, respectively, demonstrating their usefulness for predicting aspiration pneumonia. Moreover, the authors stated that the risk of silent aspiration was thought to be high when an abnormality was found in the cough test, and strategies to prevent aspiration pneumonia, such as pulse oximetry, were crucial. Perry et al. conducted a randomized controlled trial of cough test for dysphagia in 311 acute stroke patients [41] and developed the Dysphagia in Stroke Protocol (DiSP), a standardized management protocol based on a previous study showing that pneumonia was not reduced in patients who underwent a cough test [42]. They then investigated the changes in clinical outcomes after using DiSP in patients with acute stroke ($n = 432$). DiSP is a protocol in which patients who have passed the cough test proceed to the evaluation of oral intake, and patients who have failed the cough test immediately undergo a videofluoroscopic swallow study (VFSS) without oral intake. The study results of the study showed that the incidence of aspiration pneumonia after DiSP was 10%, regardless of the cough test, which was significantly lower than the 28% observed prior to using DiSP. Nevertheless, the mortality rate of patients who developed pneumonia was only slightly reduced. Thus, to reduce pneumonia-related mortality, the authors concluded that proper management of patients with silent and dominant aspiration is more important than simply identifying patients with potential aspiration.

In summary, the WST achieves various levels of sensitivity and specificity as described in the literature, but it is well known that the WST may overlook silent aspiration as it evaluates by airway response and voice changes. Therefore, further research is needed to establish the most effective combination of screening tests to detect silent aspiration. In addition, management to avoid the onset of pneumonia, such as oral care, is important for preventing pneumonia.

4. Mann Assessment of Swallowing Ability

The Mann Assessment of Swallowing Ability (MASA) was developed by the American speech therapist Mann and colleagues to evaluate swallowing dysfunction in acute stroke patients [43]. As a clinical assessment tool rather than a screening test for dysphagia, the MASA can quantify the risk of aspiration in a bedside setting using the following 24 endpoints: general patient examination (alertness, cooperation, auditory comprehension, aphasia, apraxia, and dysarthria); the oral preparation phase (saliva, lip seal, tongue movement, tongue strength, tongue coordination, oral preparation, respiration, and respiratory rate for swallowing); the oral phase (gag reflex, palatal movement, bolus clearance, and oral transit time); and the pharyngeal phase (cough reflex, voluntary cough, voice, tracheostomy, pharyngeal phase, and pharyngeal response). Each endpoint of the MASA is evaluated on a scale of 5 or 10 points, with a total score of 200 points. A lower score for each endpoint indicates a higher severity of dysphagia, and the suspicion of dysphagia or aspiration can be determined from the total score of each endpoint. In acute stroke patients, dysphagia is suspected with a total MASA score of 177 points or lower, and aspiration is suspected with a total MASA score of 169 points or lower.

The sensitivity and specificity of the MASA for predicting of dysphagia in stroke patients were reported to be 73% and 89%, respectively, in comparison with VFSS. In addition, the sensitivity and specificity of the MASA for the prediction of aspiration were reported to be 93% and 63%, respectively [23]. The MASA is currently used for various diseases, and its sensitivity and specificity for evaluation in a mixed disease population were 39.6% and 59%, respectively, when VFSS was used as the gold standard [24]. Antonios et al. statistically reviewed the original MASA data and identified items important for developing a clinical assessment tool that could be used more rapidly and accurately [25]. As a result, they devised a modified MASA (mMASA), a simplified version of the MASA, to utilize highly distinguishable items. The mMASA showed a sensitivity of 87–92% and a specificity of 84.2–86.3% in predicting dysphagia with respect to the original MASA (Table 1).

As mentioned above, the MASA was developed to evaluate the eating and swallowing dysfunction in acute stroke patients, and the cut-off value for aspiration was set to 170 points. In addition, of the 24 items, 12 items of "alertness, cooperation, auditory comprehension, respiration, dysphasia, dysarthria, saliva, tongue movement, tongue strength, gag, voluntary cough, and palate" are specified in the mMASA. Therefore, a study examined the calculation of the cut-off value of the MASA suitable for the elderly requiring nursing care for various diseases and the usefulness of the endpoints of the MASA [44]. In this study, based on the total score of the MASA and the results of the fiberoptic endoscopic swallow study (FEES), a cut-off value for aspiration was 122 points with a sensitivity and specificity of 75% and 90%, respectively. In addition, the sensitivity and specificity were 90% and 33%, respectively, when the cut-off value of 170 points for acute stroke patients was used. This indicates that the number of false-negative diagnoses increased when the original cut-off value was used for the elderly requiring nursing care. In addition, of the 24 items evaluated in the MASA, the following 8 items were shown to be potentially useful for evaluating the eating and swallowing functions of the elderly requiring nursing care:

6 items of "cooperation, oral preparation, oral transit time, cough reflex, pharyngeal phase, and pharyngeal response" that do not require the execution of instructed movements, as well as 2 items of "tongue strength and tongue coordination" which have been associated with sarcopenic dysphagia [31,45].

Research on MASA and Pneumonia

The MASA has been used to predict pneumonia in hospitalized patients. Mitani et al. conducted a retrospective observational study to determine whether the onset of pneumonia could be predicted in 393 hospitalized patients (average age 79.2 ± 11.4 years). The etiologies of the participants were as follows: Parkinson's disease ($n = 111$), multiple cerebral infarctions ($n = 73$), cerebral infarction ($n = 57$), orthopedic diseases ($n = 23$), disuse ($n = 10$), cerebral hemorrhage ($n = 9$), subarachnoid hemorrhage ($n = 6$), chronic obstructive lung disease ($n = 3$), neuromuscular disease (excluding Parkinson's disease; $n = 66$) and others ($n = 35$)) [46]. The follow-up period was 365 days, and the items of the MASA, Functional Independence Measure (FIM), and Controlling Nutrition Status (CONUT) were investigated. The results showed that 102 patients developed pneumonia and that FIM and MASA scores were significantly lower in the group with pneumonia than in the group without pneumonia, while the average age and the CONUT scores were higher in the group with pneumonia than in the group without pneumonia. The cut-off MASA score was 170.5 points, with a sensitivity and specificity of 70% and 83%, respectively, and the authors stated that the MASA might be a useful tool for predicting the onset of pneumonia. Chojin et al. conducted a prospective cohort study of 153 elderly hospitalized patients with pneumonia who were evaluated by a speech-language pathologist using the MASA (average age of 85.4 ± 9.9 years) [47]. In this study, a multivariate analysis showed that a MASA score of 169 points or lower was an independent risk factor for recurrence of pneumonia within 30 days and mortality after 6 months. Therefore, the authors stated that, for patients with a low MASA score, it is important to start oral care and appropriately evaluate and support various aspects of life, such as diet, posture during meals, mealtime, and degree of care.

The MASA can be performed with minimal items, such as a penlight, a tongue depressor, and test foods that require mastication. With its low invasiveness, the MASA can be performed by speech therapists and nurses, in addition to doctors, and is considered useful for temporal evaluations, such as regular evaluation to predict the onset of pneumonia and evaluation of training effects. In patients with a low MASA score, it is important to prevent pneumonia by intervening early in dysphagia. However, the MASA, which focuses on indirect endpoints of swallowing, requires additional tests to propose a food style suitable for the patient.

5. Gugging Swallowing Screen

One of the screening tests that can recommend a food style is the Gugging Swallowing Screen (GUSS), which was developed at the Landesklinikum Donauregion Gugging in collaboration with Danube University Krems in Austria to evaluate the severity of dysphagia and the risk of aspiration in acute stroke patients. The GUSS is currently used to evaluate dysphagia in various diseases, and it has been translated into multiple languages and is widely used internationally [48]. The GUSS is divided into an indirect swallowing test in Part 1 and a direct swallowing test in Part 2, consisting of three subtests, all of which must be performed in succession. The direct swallowing test starts with semisolid foods, which are considered less challenging for acute stroke patients, and gradually step up to more challenging test items, such as liquid and solid test foods. In addition, the liquid swallowing subtest of the GUSS uses a titration method in which the amount of water is gradually increased in steps of 3, 5, 10, 20, and 50 mL. The subtests are evaluated based on points, with higher points indicating a better grade. A maximum of five points is given in each subtest, with a total of 20 points over four subtests, and a patient must achieve the maximum score of 5 points to advance to the next subtest. Based on the score, the following diet is recommended: a regular diet for the maximum score of 20 points, a swallowing-adjusted diet and small amounts of liquid for 15–19 points, a baby food-like swallowing-adjusted diet in combination with an alternative nutrition method for 10–14 points, and no oral intake for 9 points or lower. In addition, consultation with a swallowing specialist and further evaluation by FEES and VFSS is recommended for patients with 19 points or lower.

Studies on the effectiveness of the GUSS have been carried out on stroke patients. In addition, the cut-off value of the GUSS was set to 14 points, and it was examined using FEES. Trapl et al. prospectively evaluated 50 acute stroke patients in an upright position of at least 60 degrees in bed and capable of recognizing the examiner's face, spoon, and texture in front of him/her at the start of GUSS [26]. They found that the GUSS had a sensitivity of 100%, a specificity of 50–69%, and a negative predictive value of 100%. Warnecke et al. examined 100 acute stroke patients using a prospective, double-blind method and reported that the GUSS screened for risk of aspiration with a high sensitivity of 96.5% and a specificity of 55.8% [27]. They also stated that low specificity was associated with the high rate of failure to complete the initial part of the GUSS in severe cases with a National Institute of Health Stroke Scale score of 15 points or higher. The effectiveness of the GUSS may vary depending on the severity of the stroke. Said Bassiouny et al. prospectively evaluated 40 acute stroke patients [28]. High sensitivity (93.7%) and high specificity (92.5%) were observed in patients who were clearly conscious and able to follow instructions (Table 1).

Research on GUSS and Pneumonia

Studies relating to GUSS and pneumonia have evaluated measures for predicting stroke-associated pneumonia (SAP) in stroke patients and their role in reducing the incidence of SAP. Quyet et al. prospectively surveyed 508 patients hospitalized within 5 days of stroke onset, which showed an incidence of SAP of 13.4% [49]. Logistic regression analysis showed that a GUSS score of 15 points or lower was associated with SAP (odds ratio 11.7, 95% confidence interval of 6.6–20.8, p-value < 0.01). The authors concluded that dysphagia was an independent risk factor for pneumonia. Dang et al. conducted a cohort study enrolling 892 acute stroke patients, which showed an incidence of SAP of 13.8% [50]. With a sensitivity and specificity of 80.5% and 80.1%, respectively, they stated that the GUSS was superior in predicting SAP. In addition, logistic regression analysis showed an odds ratio (OR) of 11.4, a 95% confidence interval of 7.4–17.5, and a p-value of < 0.01 (solid food is bread).

Regarding the decrease in the incidence of SAP, Teuschl et al. compared patients evaluated by the GUSS with those who were not evaluated, using a database containing 1394 patients hospitalized for acute stroke [51]. A total of 993 patients (71.2%) was screened by GUSS, of whom 50 (5.0%) developed SAP. The incidence of SAP in these patients was 22 (5.5%), which was comparable to that in 401 patients who were not screened. The incidence of SAP was low compared to the overall incidence in recent meta-analyses, suggesting that the GUSS was effective in preventing SAP. However, no difference was observed between the two groups, which may be because cases of extremely severe stroke, for which early testing was not possible, and very mild cases, for which pneumonia was not expected, were likely not screened, masking the positive effects of the intervention. Furthermore, they concluded that identifying patients at risk for SAP using the GUSS, including those with very mild stroke, and other management factors, such as the timing of nasogastric tube insertion, oral hygiene, and administration of antibiotics, in addition to diet therapy, were also helpful in further reducing the incidence of SAP. Sørensen et al. conducted a controlled trial in acute stroke patients, which consisted of an intervention group that received oral hygiene based on GUSS by a speech and language pathologist, a standardized care plan immediately after admission (n = 58), and a control group that received arbitrary clinical swallowing screening and oral hygiene (n = 88) [52]. The results showed that the incidence of SAP was 7% in the intervention group and 27% in the control group, and they reported that the incidence of SAP was significantly reduced by early systematic screening using the GUSS and enhanced oral hygiene (solid food is dry bread). Similarly, another study compared the incidence of SAP between the intervention group (n = 186), in which nurses performed GUSS all year round, and the control group (n = 198), in which only speech therapists performed GUSS during working hours [53]. They reported that the time from admission to GUSS was shorter in the intervention group and that the incidence of SAP was significantly lower in the intervention group (3.8%) than in the control group (11.6%). Furthermore, the intervention group had shorter hospital stays and lower short-term in-hospital mortality rates. However, another study compared the duration of systematic 10-mL WST (n = 204) with the duration of systematic GUSS administration by trained nurses (n = 140), reporting that they showed no difference of SAP or mortality [54].

Based on these results, SAP can be predicted and prevented by systematically implementing the GUSS at an early stage and examining the food style. This allows for early evaluation of the swallowing function after hospitalization, and prompt consultation with a swallowing specialist or performance with FEES and VFSS. Upon inspection of dysphagia or aspiration, the incidence of SAP is thought to be reduced. Further studies, including those on patients other than those with acute stroke, are expected to validate the effectiveness of the GUSS. A 2012 systematic review by Wilkinson et al. of bedside diagnostic tests for aspiration and predictors of pneumonia in older patients without stroke stated that the existing evidence is insufficient to support the use of bedside tests in the general elderly population A systematic review of predictors of inflammatory bowel disease stated that existing evidence was insufficient to support the use of bedside testing in the general population [55]. Currently, a scoping review protocol on the psychometric properties of tools for initial screening of oropharyngeal dysphagia in older people is underway [56].

6. Conclusions

We believe that pneumonia can be predicted by screening tests, such as the WST, MASA, and GUSS, as discussed in this review. Studies that reported the prevention of pneumonia used these screening tests in combination with DiSP, early systematic GUSS administration, or enhanced oral hygiene. Therefore, the response after predicting pneumonia by screening tests at an early stage is thought to be important for preventing pneumonia. Many studies have stated that an interdisciplinary team approach improves the efficiency and quality of treatment to prevent and reduce aspiration. However, it is difficult to identify which team approach is most effective and which type of treatment combination is the most optimal. Future intervention studies that investigate multiple factors and focus on the elderly are needed.

Author Contributions: Conceptualization, I.O. and S.E.; data curation, I.O.; writing—original draft preparation, I.O.; writing—review and editing, S.E.; visualization, I.O.; supervision, S.E.; funding acquisition, S.E. All authors have read and agreed to the published version of the manuscript.

Funding: This work was supported by the Japan Society for the Promotion of Science KAKENHI (Grant Nos. 19H03984 and 19K22821) to Satoru Ebihara.

Conflicts of Interest: The authors declare no conflict of interest.

References

1. Wirth, R.; Dziewas, R.; Beck, A.M.; Clave, P.; Hamdy, S.; Heppner, H.J.; Langmore, S.; Leischker, A.H.; Martino, R.; Pluschinski, P.; et al. Oropharyngeal dysphagia in older persons—From pathophysiology to adequate intervention: A review and summary of an international expert meeting. *Clin. Interv. Aging* **2016**, *11*, 189–208. [CrossRef]
2. International Trends in Population Aging/White Paper on Aging Society 2008 (Full Version)—Cabinet Office, Government of Japan. Available online: https://www8.cao.go.jp/kourei/whitepaper/w-2018/html/zenbun/s1_1_2.html (accessed on 14 October 2021).
3. Maeda, K.; Koga, T.; Akagi, J. Tentative nil per os leads to poor outcomes in older adults with aspiration pneumonia. *Clin. Nutr.* **2016**, *35*, 1147–1152. [CrossRef]
4. Estupiñán Artiles, C.; Regan, J.; Donnellan, C. Dysphagia screening in residential care settings: A scoping review. *Int. J. Nurs. Stud.* **2021**, *114*, 103813. [CrossRef] [PubMed]
5. De Lima, M.S.; Sassi, F.C.; De Medeiros, G.C.; Jayanthi, S.K.; De Andrade, C.R.F. Precisão diagnóstica para o risco de broncoaspiração em população heterogênea. *CoDAS* **2020**, *32*, e20190166. [CrossRef] [PubMed]

6. Schultheiss, C.; Nusser-Müller-Busch, R.; Seidl, R.O. The semisolid bolus swallow test for clinical diagnosis of oropharyngeal dysphagia: A prospective randomised study. *Eur. Arch. Oto-Rhino-Laryngol.* **2011**, *268*, 1837–1844. [CrossRef]
7. Brodsky, M.B.; Suiter, D.M.; González-Fernández, M.; Michtalik, H.J.; Frymark, T.B.; Venediktov, R.; Schooling, T. Screening Accuracy for Aspiration Using Bedside Water Swallow Tests. *Chest* **2016**, *150*, 148–163. [CrossRef]
8. Daniels, S.K.; Anderson, J.A.; Willson, P.C. Valid Items for Screening Dysphagia Risk in Patients with Stroke. *Stroke* **2012**, *43*, 892–897. [CrossRef]
9. Jiang, J.-L.; Fu, S.-Y.; Wang, W.-H.; Ma, Y.-C. Validity and reliability of swallowing screening tools used by nurses for dysphagia: A systematic review. *Tzu Chi Med. J.* **2016**, *28*, 41–48. [CrossRef]
10. Szabó, P.T.; Műhelyi, V.; Béres-Molnár, K.A.; Kovács, A.; Balogh, Z.; Folyovich, A. Dysphagiafelmérések akut stroke-ban. *Ideggyogy. Sz.* **2021**, *74*, 235–248. [CrossRef] [PubMed]
11. Park, Y.-H.; Bang, H.L.; Han, H.-R.; Chang, H.-K. Dysphagia Screening Measures for Use in Nursing Homes: A Systematic Review. *J. Korean Acad. Nurs.* **2015**, *45*, 1–13. [CrossRef] [PubMed]
12. Park, K.D.; Kim, T.H.; Lee, S.H. The Gugging Swallowing Screen in dysphagia screening for patients with stroke: A systematic review. *Int. J. Nurs. Stud.* **2020**, *107*, 103588. [CrossRef]
13. Perren, A.; Zürcher, P.; Schefold, J.C. Clinical Approaches to Assess Post-extubation Dysphagia (PED) in the Critically Ill. *Dysphagia* **2019**, *34*, 475–486. [CrossRef] [PubMed]
14. Wakasugi, Y.; Tohara, H.; Hattori, F.; Motohashi, Y.; Nakane, A.; Goto, S.; Ouchi, Y.; Mikushi, S.; Takeuchi, S.; Uematsu, H. Screening Test for Silent Aspiration at the Bedside. *Dysphagia* **2008**, *23*, 364–370. [CrossRef] [PubMed]
15. Momosaki, R.; Abo, M.; Kakuda, W.; Kobayashi, K. Applicability of the Two-Step Thickened Water Test in Patients with Poststroke Dysphagia: A Novel Assessment Tool for Paste Food Aspiration. *J. Stroke Cerebrovasc. Dis.* **2013**, *22*, 817–821. [CrossRef]
16. McCullough, G.H.; Rosenbek, J.C.; Wertz, R.T.; McCoy, S.; Mann, G.; McCullough, K. Utility of Clinical Swallowing Examination Measures for Detecting Aspiration Post-Stroke. *J. Speech Lang. Hear. Res.* **2005**, *48*, 1280–1293. [CrossRef]
17. Suiter, D.M.; Leder, S.B. Clinical Utility of the 3-ounce Water Swallow Test. *Dysphagia* **2008**, *23*, 244–250. [CrossRef]
18. Zhou, Z.; Salle, J.; Daviet, J.; Stuit, A.; Nguyen, C. Combined approach in bedside assessment of aspiration risk post stroke: PASS. *Eur. J. Phys. Rehabil. Med.* **2011**, *47*, 441–446.
19. Patterson, J.M.; Hildreth, A.; McColl, E.; Carding, P.N.; Hamilton, D.; Wilson, J.A. The clinical application of the 100 mL water swallow test in head and neck cancer. *Oral Oncol.* **2011**, *47*, 180–184. [CrossRef]
20. Hey, C.; Lange, B.P.; Eberle, S.; Zaretsky, Y.; Sader, R.; Stöver, T.; Wagenblast, J. Water swallow screening test for patients after surgery for head and neck cancer: Early identification of dysphagia, aspiration and limitations of oral intake. *Anticancer Res.* **2013**, *33*, 4017–4021.
21. Somasundaram, S.; Henke, C.; Neumann-Haefelin, T.; Isenmann, S.; Hattingen, E.; Lorenz, M.W.; Singer, O.C. Dysphagia Risk Assessment in Acute Left-Hemispheric Middle Cerebral Artery Stroke. *Cerebrovasc. Dis.* **2014**, *37*, 217–222. [CrossRef]
22. The Value of Bedside Tests in Dysphagia Evaluation—ScienceDirect. Available online: https://www.sciencedirect.com/science/article/pii/S2090074014000565?via%3Dihub (accessed on 14 October 2021).
23. Mann, G.; Hankey, G.; Cameron, D. Swallowing Disorders following Acute Stroke: Prevalence and Diagnostic Accuracy. *Cerebrovasc. Dis.* **2000**, *10*, 380–386. [CrossRef] [PubMed]
24. González-Fernández, M.; Sein, M.T.; Palmer, J.B. Clinical Experience Using the Mann Assessment of Swallowing Ability for Identification of Patients at Risk for Aspiration in a Mixed-Disease Population. *Am. J. Speech-Lang. Pathol.* **2011**, *20*, 331–336. [CrossRef]
25. Antonios, N.; Carnaby-Mann, G.; Crary, M.; Miller, L.; Hubbard, H.; Hood, K.; Sambandam, R.; Xavier, A.; Silliman, S. Analysis of a Physician Tool for Evaluating Dysphagia on an Inpatient Stroke Unit: The Modified Mann Assessment of Swallowing Ability. *J. Stroke Cerebrovasc. Dis.* **2010**, *19*, 49–57. [CrossRef]
26. Trapl, M.; Enderle, P.; Nowotny, M.; Teuschl, Y.; Matz, K.; Dachenhausen, A.; Brainin, M. Dysphagia Bedside Screening for Acute-Stroke Patients. *Stroke* **2007**, *38*, 2948–2952. [CrossRef] [PubMed]
27. Warnecke, T.; Im, S.; Kaiser, C.; Hamacher, C.; Oelenberg, S.; Dziewas, R. Aspiration and dysphagia screening in acute stroke—The Gugging Swallowing Screen revisited. *Eur. J. Neurol.* **2017**, *24*, 594–601. [CrossRef]
28. Bassiouny, S.E.S. Assessment of Dysphagia in Acute Stroke Patients by the Gugging Swallowing screen. *Glob. J. Otolaryngol.* **2017**, *9*. [CrossRef]
29. Suiter, D.M.; Sloggy, J.; Leder, S.B. Validation of the Yale Swallow Protocol: A Prospective Double-Blinded Videofluoroscopic Study. *Dysphagia* **2014**, *29*, 199–203. [CrossRef] [PubMed]
30. Denuit, C.; Delcourt, S.; Poncelet, M.; Dardenne, N.; Lagier, A.; Gillain, S. Benefits and limitations of geriatric dysphagia screening tools. *Rev. Med. Liege* **2021**, *76*, 280–286.
31. Chen, Y.-C.; Chen, P.-Y.; Wang, Y.-C.; Wang, T.-G.; Han, D.-S. Decreased swallowing function in the sarcopenic elderly without clinical dysphagia: A cross-sectional study. *BMC Geriatr.* **2020**, *20*, 419. [CrossRef]
32. Fujishima, I.; Fujiu-Kurachi, M.; Arai, H.; Hyodo, M.; Kagaya, H.; Maeda, K.; Mori, T.; Nishioka, S.; Oshima, F.; Ogawa, S.; et al. Sarcopenia and dysphagia: Position paper by four professional organizations. *Geriatr. Gerontol. Int.* **2019**, *19*, 91–97. [CrossRef]
33. Miki, Y.; Makuuchi, R.; Honda, S.; Tokunaga, M.; Tanizawa, Y.; Bando, E.; Kawamura, T.; Yurikusa, T.; Tanuma, A.; Terashima, M. Prospective phase II study evaluating the efficacy of swallow ability screening tests and pneumonia prevention using a team approach for elderly patients with gastric cancer. *Gastric Cancer* **2018**, *21*, 353–359. [CrossRef]

34. Ebersole, B.; Lango, M.; Ridge, J.; Handorf, E.; Farma, J.; Clark, S.; Jamal, N. Dysphagia Screening for Pneumonia Prevention in a Cancer Hospital: Results of a Quality/Safety Initiative. *Otolaryngol. Head Neck Surg.* **2020**, *162*, 220–229. [CrossRef]
35. Oguchi, N.; Yamamoto, S.; Terashima, S.; Arai, R.; Sato, M.; Ikegami, S.; Horiuchi, H. The modified water swallowing test score is the best predictor of postoperative pneumonia following extubation in cardiovascular surgery: A Retrospective Cohort Study. *Medicine* **2021**, *100*, e24478. [CrossRef]
36. Grimm, J.C.; Magruder, J.T.; Ohkuma, R.; Dungan, S.P.; Hayes, A.; Vose, A.K.; Orlando, M.; Sussman, M.S.; Cameron, D.E.; Whitman, G.J.R. A Novel Risk Score to Predict Dysphagia After Cardiac Surgery Procedures. *Ann. Thorac. Surg.* **2015**, *100*, 568–574. [CrossRef]
37. Britton, D.; Roeske, A.; Ennis, S.K.; Benditt, J.O.; Quinn, C.; Graville, D. Utility of Pulse Oximetry to Detect Aspiration: An Evidence-Based Systematic Review. *Dysphagia* **2018**, *33*, 282–292. [CrossRef]
38. Lagarde, M.L.J.; Kamalski, D.M.A.; van den Engel-Hoek, L. The reliability and validity of cervical auscultation in the diagnosis of dysphagia: A systematic review. *Clin. Rehabilit.* **2016**, *30*, 199–207. [CrossRef]
39. Donohue, C.; Mao, S.; Sejdić, E.; Coyle, J.L. Tracking Hyoid Bone Displacement During Swallowing Without Videofluoroscopy Using Machine Learning of Vibratory Signals. *Dysphagia* **2021**, *36*, 259–269. [CrossRef] [PubMed]
40. Nakamori, M.; Imamura, E.; Kuwabara, M.; Ayukawa, T.; Tachiyama, K.; Kamimura, T.; Hayashi, Y.; Matsushima, H.; Funai, M.; Mizoue, T.; et al. Simplified cough test can predict the risk for pneumonia in patients with acute stroke. *PLoS ONE* **2020**, *15*, e0239590. [CrossRef]
41. Miles, A.; Zeng, I.S.L.; McLauchlan, H.; Huckabee, M.-L. Cough Reflex Testing in Dysphagia Following Stroke: A Randomized Controlled Trial. *J. Clin. Med. Res.* **2013**, *5*, 222–233. [CrossRef]
42. Perry, S.E.; Miles, A.; Fink, J.N.; Huckabee, M.-L. The Dysphagia in Stroke Protocol Reduces Aspiration Pneumonia in Patients with Dysphagia Following Acute Stroke: A Clinical Audit. *Transl. Stroke Res.* **2019**, *10*, 36–43. [CrossRef] [PubMed]
43. Mann, G. *MASA: The Mann Assessment of Swallowing Ability*; Thomson Learning Inc.: Clifton, NY, USA, 2002.
44. Ohira, M.; Ishida, R.; Maki, Y.; Ohkubo, M.; Sugiyama, T.; Sakayori, T.; Sato, T. Evaluation of a dysphagia screening system based on the Mann Assessment of Swallowing Ability for use in dependent older adults. *Geriatr. Gerontol. Int.* **2017**, *17*, 561–567. [CrossRef]
45. Shimizu, A.; Maeda, K.; Nagami, S.; Nagano, A.; Yamada, Y.; Shimizu, M.; Ishida, Y.; Kayashita, J.; Fujishima, I.; Mori, N.; et al. Low tongue strength is associated with oral and cough-related abnormalities in older inpatients. *Nutrition* **2021**, *83*, 111062. [CrossRef]
46. Mitani, Y.; Oki, Y.; Fujimoto, Y.; Yamaguchi, T.; Yamada, Y.; Yamada, K.; Ito, T.; Shiotani, H.; Ishikawa, A. Relationship between the Functional Independence Measure and Mann Assessment of Swallowing Ability in hospitalized patients with pneumonia. *Geriatr. Gerontol. Int.* **2018**, *18*, 1620–1624. [CrossRef]
47. Chojin, Y.; Kato, T.; Rikihisa, M.; Omori, M.; Noguchi, S.; Akata, K.; Ogoshi, T.; Yatera, K.; Mukae, H. Evaluation of the Mann Assessment of Swallowing Ability in Elderly Patients with Pneumonia. *Aging Dis.* **2017**, *8*, 420–433. [CrossRef]
48. Welcome to the Guss Blog! Gugging Swallowing Screen. 2016. Available online: https://gussgroupinternational.wordpress.com/home/ (accessed on 12 December 2021).
49. Quyet, D.; Hien, N.M.; Khan, M.X.; Pham, D.D.; Thuan, D.D.; Dang, D.M.; Hai, N.D.; Van Nam, B.; Huy, P.Q.; Mai, T.D.; et al. Risk Factors for Stroke Associated Pneumonia. *Open Access Maced. J. Med. Sci.* **2019**, *7*, 4416–4419. [CrossRef]
50. Dang, P.D.; Nguyen, M.H.; Mai, X.K.; Pham, D.D.; Dang, M.D.; Nguyen, D.H.; Bui, V.N.; Mai, D.T.; Do, N.B.; Do, D.T. A Comparison of the National Institutes of Health Stroke Scale and the Gugging Swallowing Screen in Predicting Stroke-Associated Pneumonia. *Ther. Clin. Risk Manag.* **2020**, *16*, 445–450. [CrossRef]
51. Teuschl, Y.; Trapl, M.; Ratajczak, P.; Matz, K.; Dachenhausen, A.; Brainin, M. Systematic dysphagia screening and dietary modifications to reduce stroke-associated pneumonia rates in a stroke-unit. *PLoS ONE* **2018**, *13*, e0192142. [CrossRef]
52. Sørensen, R.T.; Rasmussen, R.S.; Overgaard, K.; Lerche, A.; Johansen, A.M.; Lindhardt, T. Dysphagia Screening and Intensified Oral Hygiene Reduce Pneumonia After Stroke. *J. Neurosci. Nurs.* **2013**, *45*, 139–146. [CrossRef]
53. Palli, C.; Fandler, S.; Doppelhofer, K.; Niederkorn, K.; Enzinger, C.; Vetta, C.; Trampusch, E.; Schmidt, R.; Fazekas, F.; Gattringer, T. Early Dysphagia Screening by Trained Nurses Reduces Pneumonia Rate in Stroke Patients: A Clinical Intervention Study. *Stroke* **2017**, *48*, 2583–2585. [CrossRef]
54. Lopes, M.; Freitas, E.; Oliveira, M.; Dantas, E.; Azevedo, N.; Rodrigues, P.; Pinho, J.; Ferreira, C. Impact of the systematic use of the Gugging Swallowing Screen in patients with acute ischaemic stroke. *Eur. J. Neurol.* **2019**, *26*, 722–726. [CrossRef]
55. Wilkinson, A.H.; Burns, S.L.; Witham, M.D. Aspiration in older patients without stroke: A systematic review of bedside diagnostic tests and predictors of pneumonia. *Eur. Geriatr. Med.* **2012**, *3*, 145–152. [CrossRef]
56. Lauridsen, M.K.; Møller, L.B.; Pedersen, P.U. Psychometric properties of tools for initial screening for oropharyngeal dysphagia in older people: A scoping review protocol. *JBI Évid. Synth.* **2021**, *19*, 1948–1953. [CrossRef]

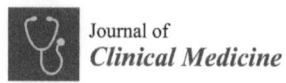

Review

Systematic Review of Incidence Studies of Pneumonia in Persons with Spinal Cord Injury

Anja Maria Raab [1,2,*], Gabi Mueller [1], Simone Elsig [3], Simon C. Gandevia [4,5], Marcel Zwahlen [6], Maria T. E. Hopman [7] and Roger Hilfiker [3]

1. Clinical Trial Unit, Swiss Paraplegic Centre, 6207 Nottwil, Switzerland; gabi.mueller@paraplegia.ch
2. Department of Health Professions, Bern University of Applied Sciences, 3008 Bern, Switzerland
3. School of Health Sciences Valais, Physiotherapy, University of Applied Sciences and Arts Western Switzer Land Valais, 1950 Sion, Switzerland; simone.elsig@hevs.ch (S.E.); roger.hilfiker@hevs.ch (R.H.)
4. Neuroscience Research Australia, Randwick 2031, Australia; s.gandevia@neura.edu.au
5. School of Medical Sciences, University of New South Wales, Sydney 2052, Australia
6. Institute of Social and Preventive Medicine, University of Bern, 3012 Bern, Switzerland; marcel.zwahlen@ispm.unibe.ch
7. Department of Physiology, Radboud University Nijmegen, 6525 Nijmegen, The Netherlands; maria.hopman@radboudumc.nl
* Correspondence: anja.raab@bfh.ch

Abstract: Pneumonia continues to complicate the course of spinal cord injury (SCI). Currently, clinicians and policy-makers are faced with only limited numbers of pneumonia incidence in the literature. A systematic review of the literature was undertaken to provide an objective synthesis of the evidence about the incidence of pneumonia in persons with SCI. Incidence was calculated per 100 person-days, and meta-regression was used to evaluate the influence of the clinical setting, the level of injury, the use of mechanical ventilation, the presence of tracheostomy, and dysphagia. For the meta-regression we included 19 studies. The incidence ranged from 0.03 to 7.21 patients with pneumonia per 100 days. The main finding of this review is that we found large heterogeneity in the reporting of the incidence, and we therefore should be cautious with interpreting the results. In the multivariable meta-regression, the incidence rate ratios showed very wide confidence intervals, which does not allow a clear conclusion concerning the risk of pneumonia in the different stages after a SCI. Large longitudinal studies with a standardized reporting on risk factors, pneumonia, and detailed time under observation are needed. Nevertheless, this review showed that pneumonia is still a clinically relevant complication and pneumonia prevention should focus on the ICU setting and patients with complete tetraplegia.

Keywords: pneumonia; spinal cord injury; systematic review; incidence

1. Introduction

Pneumonia continues to complicate the course of spinal cord injury (SCI). Currently, clinicians and policy-makers are faced with only limited numbers of pneumonia incidence in the literature. Respiratory complications are one of the main comorbidities after SCI, especially among persons with cervical and high thoracic injury [1]. The underlying problem is paralysis of the respiratory muscles, which leads to poor mobilization of secretion, bacterial accumulation in the secretion, and resultant respiratory infections [1–3]. The higher the level of SCI, the greater is the risk of respiratory complications [2]. About 30% of all deaths after an SCI are due to respiratory causes, with pneumonia as the most common respiratory cause [4].

Pneumonia is defined as inflammation of the lung tissue and is usually caused by infection [5,6]. The United States Centers for Disease Control and Prevention provide an overview of causes of pneumonia [7]. Pneumonia can be caused by viruses, bacteria, and

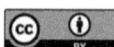

fungi. Common causes of viral pneumonia are influenza viruses, respiratory syncytial virus, and SARS-CoV-2. A common cause of bacterial pneumonia is Streptococcus [8,9]. However, clinicians are not always able to find out which pathogen caused pneumonia. Generally, the bacteria and viruses that most commonly cause pneumonia in the community are different from those in healthcare settings [7]. Diagnosis can be made by radiographic signs of parenchymal disease [6] or clinical signs such as fever, inflammatory markers or purulent tracheobronchial secretions.

Pneumonia profoundly impacts the length of hospital stay and the neurological outcome in persons with SCI [10]. Many persons with SCI, who survive acute hospitalization, die within 6.2 years after discharge [11], mainly as a result of cardiovascular (13–37%) and pulmonary diseases (9–30%) [11–13]. In patients with community-acquired pneumonia, the case fatality rate for pneumonia (7.9% within 60 days) is greater in persons with SCI compared to the general population, and hospitalizations are more frequent with increasing age, tetraplegia, and the occurrence of comorbidities [14]. Male gender, motor complete injury, presence of chest trauma and the timing of intubation are key predictors for pneumonia in SCI [10].

The risk of pneumonia is the sum of different factors such as level of injury, the clinical setting, the use of mechanical ventilation, the presence of tracheostomy, and dysphagia. The higher the level of spinal-cord damage, the more severe are the respiratory impairment [15] and the risk of pneumonia. Respiratory dysfunction in SCI can be considered in 2 phases: (1) the initial phase immediately following the injury and the year thereafter, and (2) the chronic phase during the rest of the life of the affected individual [16]. Early after an injury, a reduction in lung compliance occurs, with reduced lung volumes and changes in the mechanical properties of the lung [16]. Brown et al. described an improvement of respiratory function with time depending on the level and completeness of the injury, the extent of the spontaneous recovery, and other factors [16]. Thus, the time post injury and the setting play an important role in the development of pneumonia. Patients affected by pneumonia can be admitted to ICUs independently by the setting where the infection has been acquired [17]. However, frequently pneumonia can develop in patients already in an ICU, especially in those requiring mechanical ventilation [17].

In persons with severe paralysis, the risk of dysphagia is increased, particularly in the first weeks after injury [18]. Mechanical ventilation and prolonged tracheostomy further increase the risk of pneumonia [19,20]. Shem et al. reported that 75% of spinal cord injured patients with dysphagia developed pneumonia compared to 29% without dysphagia [19]. Martin et al. showed that pneumonia is significantly associated with the need for a tracheostomy in 67% of patients with SCI [21].

A formal incidence of pneumonia in persons with SCI is still missing and, to our knowledge, this is the first systematic review of the incidence of pneumonia in the SCI population. Incidence of a disease indicates the number of new cases within a time period in a population. Systematic reviews of prevalence and incidence data are becoming increasingly important as decision-makers realize their usefulness in informing policy and practice [22]. Accurate estimates of the true incidence of pneumonia are also of value in improving the understanding and awareness in an SCI population and in planning diagnostic and intervention services. We hypothesized that the risk of pneumonia may be influenced by various factors such as the clinical setting, the level of injury, the use of mechanical ventilation, the presence of a tracheostomy, and the presence of dysphagia. Therefore, a systematic review of the literature was undertaken to provide an objective synthesis of the evidence about the incidence of pneumonia in persons with SCI using five covariates: clinical setting, the level of injury, use of mechanical ventilation, presence of tracheostomy, and dysphagia.

2. Materials and Methods

We conducted a systematic review and meta-regression of incidence studies of the incidence of pneumonia in SCI. The review was guided by the recommendations provided for Meta-analysis of Observational Studies in Epidemiology (MOOSE) and guidelines for undertaking systematic reviews of incidence and prevalence studies [23,24]. The review was registered with the International Prospective Register of Systematic Reviews (PROSPERO 2019 CRD42019129048).

2.1. Types of Studies

We considered all types of studies for inclusion, except case studies.

2.2. Literature Searches

A variety of sources were used to find relevant publications, including PubMed, EMBASE, MEDLINE (Ovid) and the Cochrane Central Register of Controlled Trials (CENTRAL) databases. Search terms and the combination of exploded Medical Subject Heading/Emtree terms using "or" and "and" per database specification are provided in Supplementary File S1. One review author (AMR) designed this search strategy in collaboration with an experienced health librarian. A systematic and comprehensive search was scheduled on 20 March 2019 with a final update on 12 May 2020. We also searched the reference lists of relevant papers and literature reviews by hand. We contacted study authors to acquire information that was not included in their articles. Additionally, we contacted experts in the field to find all publications that matched our inclusion criteria. Initially we applied no date, language or publication restrictions. The search strategy for the six databases is provided in Supplementary File S1. However, three papers in Chinese, Danish, and Icelandic could not be translated and they were not included in the analysis. No other studies required translation into English. Papers with low incidence may be under-represented in our final list of publications.

Eligibility Criteria

We included studies involving male and female patients with a primary diagnosis of traumatic or non-traumatic SCI, American Spinal Injury Association Impairment Scale (AIS) A–D, right and left motor level between C1-L5, both acute and chronic. The participants were 18 years of age and over. In those studies with missing information about the AIS grade, we contacted the authors of the study. For those who gave no answer we used the following definition: "complete" SCI indicates AIS A in which no motor or sensory function is preserved, and "incomplete" SCI indicates an AIS B,C,D in which sensory but no or partial motor function is preserved [25]. In the included studies, only the term "pneumonia" was used, and the causes and types of pneumonia were not specifically defined. Therefore, analysis among different types of pneumonia was not possible.

Studies on patients with progressive neurological diseases such as multiple sclerosis, poliomyelitis or amyotrophic lateral sclerosis were excluded as well as studies on patients with mental disorders, patients taking bronchodilators or any other medication that influences respiration at the time of assessment. We also did not include studies that investigated pneumonia caused by the recently discovered coronavirus with the outbreak in China in December 2019 and the ensuing pandemic.

Full-text, peer-reviewed studies were required to report data on incidence of pneumonia in persons with SCI. Studies could be conducted in the hospital or community setting.

2.3. Study Records

The search results were collated in an EndNote X8 database (Clarivate Analytics, Philadelphia, PA, USA). Duplicates were removed before search results were analyzed. Two review authors (A.M.R., S.E.) independently assessed the titles and abstracts to identify potentially relevant articles by using the Covidence systematic review software (Veritas Health Innovation, Melbourne, Australia). After initial screening, the two review authors independently assessed the full texts of the retrieved articles for compliance with the eligibility criteria. Disagreement was resolved by discussion. In cases when no decision could be made by consensus, a third author (G.M.) was consulted for discussion until agreement could be reached. A PRISMA flow chart of the study selection procedure was created (Figure 1).

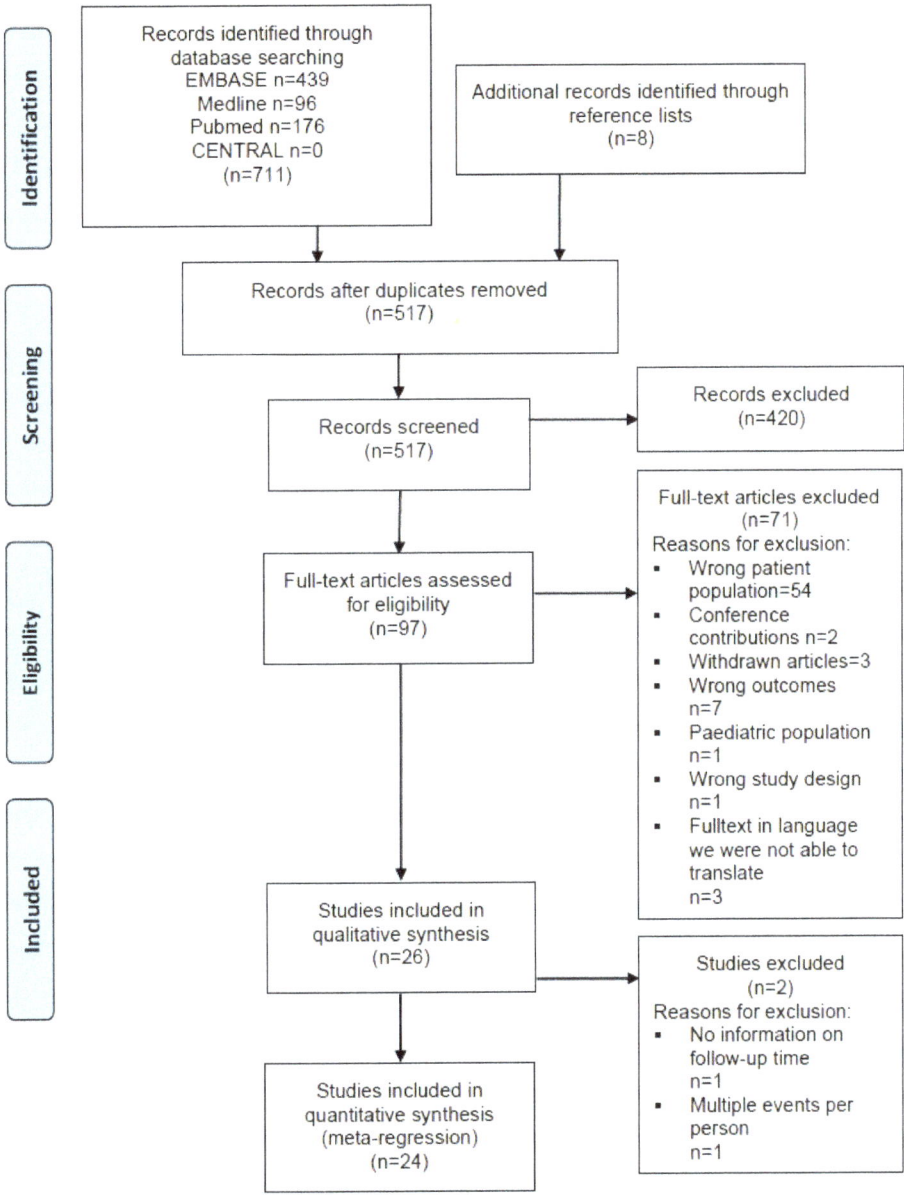

Figure 1. PRISMA flow diagram. Systematic review of incidence studies of pneumonia in persons with spinal cord injury.

2.4. Data Extraction

Methods and population characteristics reported across studies were selected for data extraction. One review author (A.M.R.) extracted and coded data from included studies by using a predefined form. A second review author (R.H.) checked the extracted data. The second review author consulted the first one in cases where there was disagreement to find a consensus. The following items were extracted: year of publication, country, design of study, sample size, clinical setting, age, sex, AIS grade, level of injury, length of hospital stay, use of mechanical ventilation, length of observation, and the incidence of pneumonia.

2.5. Data Processing

We calculated incidence rates per 100 person-days based on the number of events divided by the total exposure time in days. Because most of the studies only reported overall follow-up time and not the exact time at risk to develop pneumonia, we estimated the time at risk by taking the mean follow-up time in days for patients without pneumonia and by taking half of the mean follow-up time in days for the patients with pneumonia to adjust for the reduced time at risk in persons with a pneumonia (i.e., the person stops being at risk when diagnosed with a pneumonia) [26]. The time at risk was then multiplied by the number of participants in the study. We only considered cases with pneumonia and not episodes of pneumonia, i.e., each person was considered only once in the calculations. In a sensitivity analysis, we calculated a minimal follow-up time by using 0 days for the cases and a maximal follow-up time by using the full follow-up time for all patients.

2.6. Risk-of-Bias Assessment

Risks of bias were assessed for all included studies using a "Quality assessment checklist for prevalence studies" developed by Hoy et al. [27]. The tool consists of 10 questions, and each question can be answered as "yes", defined as low risk of bias or "no", defined as high risk of bias. The quality assessment questions addressed external validity (items 1–4) and internal validity (items 5–10) (Supplementary File S2). We selected the five most important items for the aims of our study (items 2, 4, 6, 7, 10). We decided for a conservative procedure that the worst item out of these five items was decisive for the rating of the whole study. Uncertainties in rating of the risk of bias were resolved by discussion with two further authors (R.H., G.M.). The full risk-of-bias assessment is shown in Supplementary File S3. We planned to perform sensitivity analyses comparing results from studies with a high risk of bias compared to studies with low risk of bias within the subgroups.

2.7. Data Synthesis

The incidence rates were used to calculate pooled incidence rates per subgroup (i.e., for each combination of the study characteristics) with a random-effects meta-analysis and were used to perform a meta-regression to provide the incidence-rate ratios for the independent variables: Setting, Level of Injury, Ventilation, Tracheostomy, and Dysphagia [28]. Five categorical variables were used to create the subgroups and as independent variables in the univariable and multivariable regression models: Setting (Acute, ICU, Rehabilitation, Post-Rehabilitation, Long-Term Ventilated, and Mixed), Level of Injury (studies with only persons with paraplegia, studies with only persons with tetraplegia, studies where more than 50% but less than 100% of the persons had paraplegia, studies where more than 50% but less than 100% of the persons had tetraplegia, and "mixed" for studies where the proportion of persons with paraplegia or tetraplegia was not reported), Ventilation (Not Ventilated or No Information, Ventilated, and Mixed), Tracheostomy (No, Yes, Mixed), Dysphagia (Not Mentioned, No, Yes). The categorical variable dysphagia was not entered in the multivariable meta-regression because of the low number ($n = 2$) of included studies with information on dysphagia.

Settings were divided into ICU, acute phase, rehabilitation phase, post-rehabilitation phase and mixed setting, in which the first three settings are linked to hospital-acquired pneumonia and post-rehabilitation is linked to community-acquired pneumonia. Mechanical ventilation means ventilation through a tracheostomy or an endotracheal tube [29]. Dysphagia is commonly diagnosed by a swallow evaluation at the bedside, a flexible fiberoptic endoscopy evaluation of swallowing, or a videofluoroscopic swallow study [30]. Dummy variables were created, and the category with the hypothesized lowest incidence was chosen as the reference category. The meta-regression was performed with a Poisson regression with a random intercept, which corresponds to a random effects meta-regression. Details on this method can be found here [31,32]. Statistical heterogeneity was evaluated using tau2 and the I^2 statistic. Tau2 is between study variance of the incidence rates, and I2 describes the proportion of variation in incidence estimates that is due to genuine variation rather than sampling error. Values for I^2 of 50% or greater were considered to show substantial heterogeneity [33,34]. Analyses were performed with Stata, version 17 and R (R Foundation for Statistical Computing, Vienna, Austria) and the packages meta [35] and metafor [36].

3. Results

3.1. Studies Identified

Literature searches identified 719 records, including duplicates. Figure 1 displays the flow of the inclusion of records. After exclusion through comparisons of titles and abstracts against inclusion criteria, 97 records were identified for detailed examination. In total, 71 records were excluded (Supplementary File S4) with the reasons listed in Figure 1. The main reason was that in 54 studies the wrong patient population was examined (Figure 1). Mainly, data for the sub-analyses for the SCI population were missing and therefore the numbers for incidence of pneumonia could not be used for our analyses.

Finally, 24 records met inclusion criteria, and 19 studies could be included in the analyses for the incidence rates and incidence rate ratios. Of the 24 included studies, only 2 designed their study specifically to report on incidence of pneumonia [37,38]. The study sample sizes ranged from 14 to 18,693 (median = 90), and the studies were published between 2001 and 2020 and carried out in Europe ($n = 7$), Asia ($n = 4$) and the U.S. ($n = 13$). Of these 24 studies, 12 studies were prospective. Table 1 describes the study characteristics.

3.2. Risk of Bias

Supplementary File S3 is a tabular display of the overall risk-of-bias assessment. Of the 24 included papers, all studies were rated as having a high risk of bias; therefore, we did not undertake a risk-of-bias sensitivity analysis.

3.3. Incidence Rates per 100 Person-Days and Incidence-Rate Ratios

Meta-regression of 19 studies reporting on 34 study samples was conducted. Because Raab et al. and Smith et al. did not report cases per time units, both studies were excluded from the meta-regression. The study from McKinley et al. from 2002 and two studies from Shem et al. from 2011 and 2012 were also excluded because the use of patients in different studies is quite likely. Only the latest studies were included in the analyses to ensure that each patient is only included once in our analyses.

Figure 2 shows the incidence rates for each study and pooled for each subgroup. The incidence rates ranged from 0.06 to 3.98 per 100 person-days for the acute setting, from 0.27 to 7.21 per 100 person-days for the ICU setting, from 0 to 1.84 per 100 person-days for the rehabilitation setting, and from 0.03 to 0.96 for the post-rehabilitation setting. Figure 2 also shows that the heterogeneity remains high, even when subgroups are built with the combination of setting, level of injury, ventilation, tracheostomy, and dysphagia (high I2 in most subgroups).

Table 1. Characteristics of 24 included studies with 34 subgroups.

Citation	Year of Publication	Country	Type of Study	Sample Size (n)	Setting	Mean Age (±SD)	Sex Male(%)	SCI Classification Using AIS (%)	SCI Level of Injury (%)	Mechanical Ventilator Depen-Dency (%)
Choi et al. [39] Early Tracheostomy	2013	Korea	retro-spective	10	ICU	54 ± 14	90	A 20 B 20 C 60 D 0	Tetra 100	70
Choi et al. [39] Late Tracheostomy	2013	Korea	retrospective	11	ICU	46 ± 17	91	A 55 B 9 C 27 D 9	Tetra 100	100
Citak et al. [40] Heterotopic Ossification	2012	Germany	pro-spective	132	Mixed	43 ± N.M.	84	A 83 B,C,D 17	Tetra 55 Para 45	N.M.
Citak et al. [40] No Heterotopic Ossification	2012	Germany	pro-spective	132	Mixed	49 ± N.M.	77	A 46 B,C,D 54	Tetra 49 Para 51	N.M.
Fenton et al. [41] High Tidal	2016	USA	pro-spective	16	ICU	39 ± 13	88	A,B,C 100	Tetra 100	100
Fenton et al. [41] Low Tidal	2016	USA	pro-spective	17	ICU	27 ± 7	65	A,B,C 100	Tetra 100	100
Fussenich et al. [42]	2018	Germany	retro-spective	165	ICU	57 ± 17	79	A 46 B 12 C 32 D 11	Tetra 82 Para 19	100
Garcia-Leoni et al. [37]	2010	Spain	pro-spective	100	LT-Ventilated	49 ± 17	75	N.M.	Tetra 58 (missing data N.M.)	100
Hatton et al. [43] HighTidal Volume	2020	USA	retro-spective	22	ICU	40 (27–51)	77	A 73 B,C,D 27	Tetra 100	100
Hatton et al. [43] Standard Tidal Voluma	2020	USA	retro-spective	159	ICU	53 (35–70)	79	A 38 B,C,D 62	Tetra 100	100

Table 1. *Cont.*

Citation	Year of Publication	Country	Type of Study	Sample Size (n)	Setting	Mean Age (±SD)	Sex Male(%)	SCI Classification Using AIS (%)	SCI Level of Injury (%)	Mechanical Ventilator Depen-Dency (%)
Ito et al. [44] Mpss	2009	Japan	pro-spective	38	ICU	55 ± N.M.	79	A 26 B 11 C 29 D 34	Tetra 100	N.M.
Ito et al. [44] Non-Mpss	2009	Japan	pro-spective	41	ICU		80	A 27 B 27 C 29 D 17	Tetra 100	N.M.
Kamiya et al. [45] G-Csf	2015	Japan	retro-spective	28	Acute	58 (38–72)	75	A 7 B 14 C 29 D 50	Tetra 100	N.M.
Kamiya et al. [45] Mpss	2015	Japan	retro-spective	34	Acute	61 (18–85)	79	A 26 B 9 C 32 D 32	Tetra 97 Unclear 3	N.M.
* McKinley et al. [46]	2004	USA	retro-spective	654	Acute	38 ± 16	79	A 49 B,C,D 51	Tetra 55 Para 45	N.M.
McKinley et al. [47] Non-Traumatic	2002	USA	pro-spective	38	Acute	55 ± 14	50	A 5 B 29 C 34 D 31	Tetra 34 Para 66	N.M.
McKinley et al. [47] Traumatic	2002	USA	pro-spective	79	Acute	39 ± 16	87	A 46 B 22 C 18 D 15	Tetra 42 Para 58	N.M.
Medee et al. [38]	2010	France	retro-spective	14	ICU	41 ± 18	57	A,B 100	Tetra 100	64
Patel et al. [48]	2012	USA	retro-spective	20	Acute	76 ± n.m	65	A 55 B 10 C 15 D 20	Tetra 50 Para 5 Central Cord 45	N.M.

Table 1. Cont.

Citation	Year of Publication	Country	Type of Study	Sample Size (n)	Setting	Mean Age (±SD)	Sex Male(%)	SCI Classification Using AIS (%)	SCI Level of Injury (%)	Mechanical Ventilator Depen-Dency (%)
Raab et al. [49]	2016	Switzerland	retrospective	307	Mixed	53 ± 15 53 ± 18	81	A 58 B 20 C 13 D 9	N.M.	N.M.
Shem et al. [19] No Dysphagia	2011	USA	pro-spective	17	Acute	35 ± 12	71	N.M.	Tetra 100	41
Shem et al. [19] Dysphagia	2011	USA	pro-spective	12	Acute	49 ± 21	83	N.M.	Tetra 100	67
Shem et al. [20] No Dysphagia	2012	USA	pro-spective	24	Acute	36 ± 13	71	A 54 B,C,D 46	Tetra 100	46
Shem et al. [20] Dysphagia	2012	USA	pro-spective	16	Acute	51 ± 18	88	A 25 B,C,D 75	Tetra 100	88
Shem et al. [30] No Dysphagia	2019	USA	pro-spective	53	Acute	39 ± 17	79	A 47 B,C,D 53	Tetra 100	40
Shem et al. [30] Dysphagia	2019	USA	pro-spective	23	Acute	48 ± 19	91	A 35 B,C,D 65	Tetra 100	65
Smith et al. [50]	2007	USA	retrospective	18.693	Mixed	56 ± 14	98	A 24 B,C,D 27 Unknown 32	Tetra 33 Para 21 Missing 36	N.M.
Stillman et al. [51]	2017	USA	pro-spective	169	Post-Rehab	41 ± 16	79	A,B,C 48 D 50 Unknown 2	Tetra 23 Para 65 Unknown 2	N.M.
Street et al. [52]	2015	Canada	pro-spective	171	Post-Rehab	47 ± 20	81	N.M.	N.M.	N.M.
Unsal-Delialioglu et al. [53]	2010	Turkey	retrospective	392	Acute	37 ± 14	76	A 52 B 11 C 19 D 18	N.M.	N.M.
# Wahman et al. [54] Para	2019	Sweden	pro-spective	45	Acute	55 ± 17	60	A 29 B,C,D 71	Tetra 71 Para 29	Yes (number N.M.)
Younan et al. [55] Latent Coagulopathy	2016	USA	retrospective	73	ICU	39 ± 17	82	N.M.	° Tetra N.M. Para N.M.	100

Table 1. Cont.

Citation	Year of Publication	Country	Type of Study	Sample Size (n)	Setting	Mean Age (±SD)	Sex Male(%)	SCI Classification Using AIS (%)	SCI Level of Injury (%)	Mechanical Ventilator Dependency (%)
Younan et al. [55] Admission Coagulopathy	2016	USA	retrospective	88	ICU	39 ± 20	81	N.M.	° Tetra N.M. Para N.M.	100
Younan et al. [55] No Coagulopathy	2016	USA	retrospective	126	Rehab	44 ± 16	82	N.M.	° Tetra N.M.Para N.M.	100
Yu et al. [56] Successful Weaning	2015	Taiwan	retrospective	54	ICU	49 ± 19	83	∞ A 34 B 10 C 10 D 4 Unknown 43	Tetra 100	100
Yu et al. [56] Unsuccessful Weaning	2015	Taiwan	retrospective	19	ICU	64 ± 17	84	∞ A 34 B 10 C 10 D 4 Unknown 43	Tetra 100	100
Vitaz et al. [57] No Pathway	2001	USA	retrospective	22	ICU	34 ± 10	N.M.	N.M.	Tetra 86 Para 14	Yes (number N.M.)
Vitaz et al. [57] Pathway	2001	USA	prospective	36	ICU	33 ± 15	N.M.	N.M.	Tetra 89 Para 11	Yes (number N.M.)

ASIA = American Spinal Injury Association; CI = Confidence Interval; Gcf = granulocyte colonystimulating factor; Mpss = methylprednisolone sodium succinate; N.M. = not mentioned in study; Para = Paraplegia; SCI = Spinal Cord Injury; Tetra = Tetraplegia. All numbers are rounded up or down to a full turn-out. Mechanical ventilation: N.M.—this means that in the study it is not mentioned whether the participants needed mechanical ventilation or not; YES (number N.M.)—this means that in the study it is mentioned that the participants were ventilated, but the exact number of ventilated participants is not given; NO—the participants in the study were not ventilated. * McKinley et al. (2004) [46] only reported overall values. For our pneumonia analyses, we used the subgroups Overall_Acute/Overall_Rehab. # Wahman et al. (2019) [54] only reported overall values. For our pneumonia analyses, we used the subgroups Tetra/Para. ° Younan et al. (2016) [55] reported numbers higher than 100% with no reason given, and therefore we wrote N.M. ∞ Yu et al. (2015) [56] did not present a subdivision for ASIA for the subgroups Successful weaning/Unsuccessful weaning.

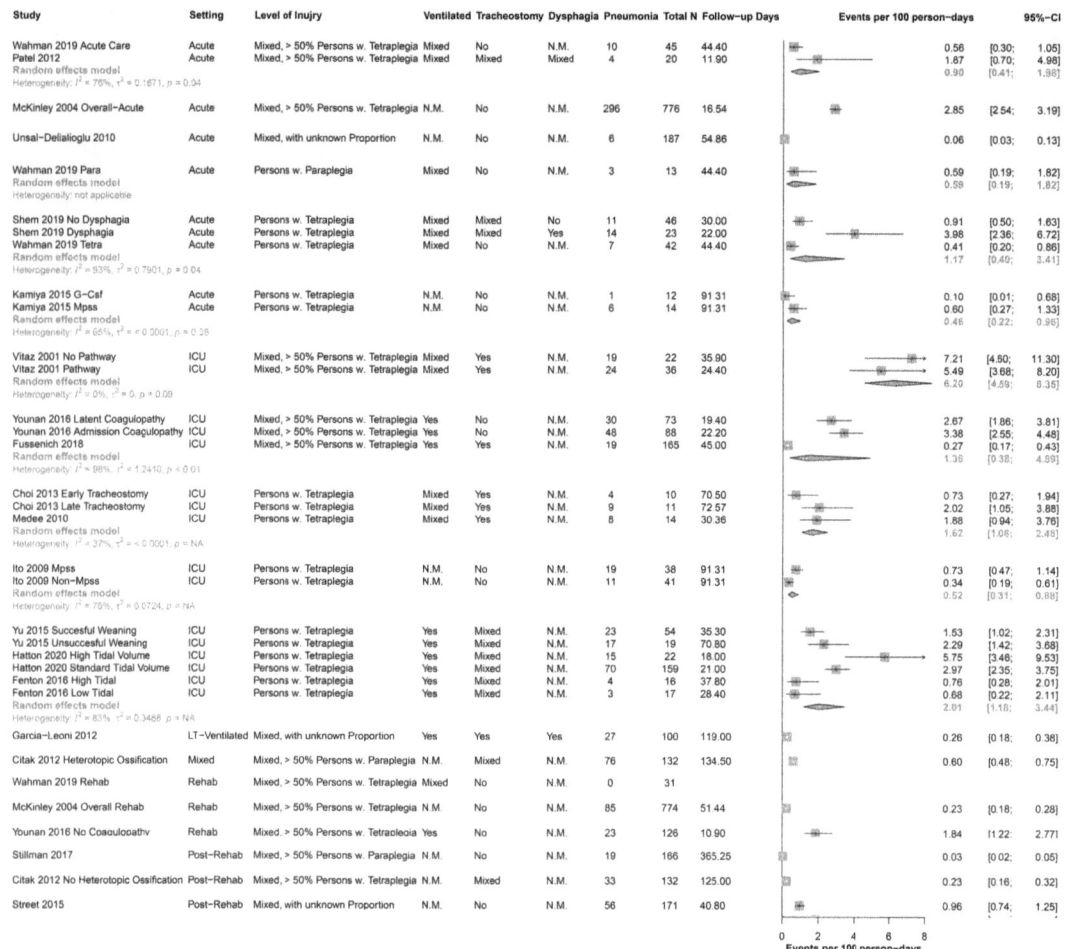

Figure 2. Forest Plot of all included study samples, without pooled results. CI = confidence interval; Fup, Follow up; G-Csf, granulocyte colonystimulating factor; ICU, Intensive Care Unit; LT-Ventilated, long-term ventilated; MPSS, high-dose methylprednisolone sodium succinate; n.m., not mentioned; Para, paraplegia; Rehab, rehabilitation; Tetra, tetraplegia; Ventilation, mechanical ventilation.

Table 2 shows the univariable and multivariable incidence rate ratios. For the setting, the incidence-rate ratio was 8.20 (95% CI 2.21 to 30.39) for the ICU compared to the post-rehabilitation setting. The incidence-rate ratios for the other settings were not statistically significant. The only other significant incidence-rate ratios were for the ventilated and mixed versus the studies where no information was given for the mechanical ventilation.

In the multivariable meta-regression (adjusted for setting, level of injury, ventilation, and tracheostomy), the incidence rate was only significant for the mixed setting versus the post-rehabilitation setting (IRR 15.76, 95% Ci 1.31 to 189.45), and the studies with a mix of ventilated and non-ventilated patients versus those with no information on ventilation (IRR 5.07, 95% CI 1.58 to 16.25).

Table 2. Univariable and multivariable Meta-Regression including Setting, Level of Injury, Ventilation, Tracheostomy, and Dysphagia.

Variable	Univariable Meta-Regression			Multivariable Meta-Regression		
	Incidence Rate Ratio	95% CI	p-Value	Incidence Rate Ratio	95% CI	p-Value
Setting						
Post-Rehab (Reference)	1.00			1.00		
Acute	3.25	0.81 to 12.97	0.095	0.65	0.13 to 3.35	0.605
ICU	8.20	2.21 to 30.39	0.002	2.27	0.32 to 15.93	0.410
Long-Term Ventilation	1.33	0.12 to 14.6	0.817	0.97	0.05 to 17.64	0.983
Mixed	3.08	0.28 to 33.3	0.355	15.76	1.31 to 189.45	0.030
Rehab	3.23	0.49 to 21.41	0.224	0.75	0.1 to 5.9	0.785
Level of Injury						
Persons w. Paraplegia (Reference)	1.00					
Mixed, >50% Persons w. Paraplegia	0.28	0.02 to 4.62	0.371	0.20	0.01 to 0.01	0.296
Mixed, >50% Persons w. Tetraplegia	2.54	0.22 to 30.11	0.459	3.64	0.41 to 0.41	0.244
Persons w. Tetraplegia	2.03	0.18 to 23.46	0.571	1.93	0.21 to 0.21	0.562
Mixed, with unknown Proportion	0.49	0.03 to 7.17	0.601	1.99	0.16 to 0.16	0.596
Ventilation						
Not mentioned (Reference)	1.00					
Mixed	4.70	1.89 to 11.72	0.001	5.07	1.58 to 16.25	0.006
Ventilated	4.34	1.76 to 10.71	0.001	2.03	0.61 to 6.73	0.247
Tracheostomy						
No (Reference)	1.00					
Mixed	2.55	0.99 to 6.57	0.053	1.17	0.42 to 3.21	0.763
Yes	2.52	0.85 to 7.48	0.096	0.41	0.1 to 1.69	0.217
Dysphagia						
No (Reference)	1.00			*		
Not mentioned	0.95	0.07 to 12.18	0.968			
Mixed	1.93	0.05 to 72.32	0.722			
Yes	1.13	0.05 to 24.19	0.938			

* Too few studies with information on dysphagia (only two studies reported on dysphagia), therefore, we did not include dysphagia in the multivariable model. Incidence Rate Ratio: exp(coefficient): how many times the incidence per 100 days is higher compared to the reference category, (in multivariable analysis: controlled for all other variables).

3.4. Sensitivity Analyses

The sensitivity analyses (Supplementary File S5) with the two alternative calculations of the time under risk did not produce results that would change the conclusion.

4. Discussion

This systematic review and meta-regression of 24 studies analyzed the incidence of pneumonia in SCI. All studies had a high risk of bias with high heterogeneity, and this was evident even in the subgroup analyses. While pooled estimates of incidence would be useful to indicate the public health burden of pneumonia in SCI, we have only low confidence in our pooled estimates of the incidence, which ranged from 0.03 to 7.21 patients with pneumonia per 100 days. This low confidence results mainly because of (i) the design of the studies, which were not specifically designed to analyze the incidence of pneumonia, (ii) the reporting of the follow-up time (time at risk), (iii) the small sample sizes, (iv) the non-standardized reporting of the outcome variables and the risk factors (i.e., setting, level of injury, mechanical ventilation, tracheostomy, dysphagia), (v) not all studies had a longitudinal design, and (vi) the high risk of bias.

Despite this, our results suggest that shortly after the onset of a SCI, when the patient is in an ICU, the incidence of pneumonia was almost five times as high as in the time after subsequent discharge from the rehabilitation setting. Given that most pneumonia occurs early after the SCI (Figure 2), we propose the need for a greater focus on regular screening of pulmonary and respiratory muscle function in the ICU and implementation of potential strategies to enhance pulmonary and respiratory muscle function (e.g., physiotherapy and respiratory muscle training).

4.1. Overall Completeness of Evidence

The overall completeness of evidence with 24 identified studies appears to be sufficient to address the incidence of pneumonia in SCI, taking into account the wide 95% confidence intervals. Most studies reported the incidence of pneumonia in SCI, and a minority reported the point prevalence or the period prevalence of pneumonia. We therefore decided to focus on incidence estimates. The analyses of incidence rates had the limitation that the time under risk was not reported. For a correct follow-up time, the follow-up days should only be counted up to the diagnosis of a pneumonia, and most studies reported the overall follow-up time, i.e., including the days where a patient was already diagnosed with a pneumonia. Therefore, we had to estimate the follow-up time by adjusting the days for patients with pneumonia (i.e., we took only half of these days for cases).

4.2. Covartiates

4.2.1. Setting

The clinical setting influences the incidence of pneumonia. Rates are considerably higher among patients hospitalized in ICUs compared with those in hospital wards [29,58]. These findings are confirmed in this systematic review; the incidence of pneumonia in SCI is also highest in ICU and decreases with time post injury (Figure 2). The clinical setting varied between the studies we examined. For example, in some studies pneumonia was identified at ICU during the acute phase of SCI, and in others pneumonia was identified in the rehabilitation phase or later in the outpatient setting.

4.2.2. Level of Injury

We investigated the incidence of pneumonia according to the level of injury. We divided the level of injury into tetraplegia and paraplegia because the degree of respiratory impairment depends on the level of injury, with higher levels of injury causing greater impairment [15,59]. Generally, the incidence of pneumonia is higher in high-level tetraplegia in comparison to low-level tetraplegia and paraplegia [6]. However, one study in this review directly compared patients with tetraplegia and paraplegia with comparable personal/baseline characteristics [54] and could not confirm this statement.

4.2.3. Mechanical Ventilation

For patients receiving mechanical ventilation, the risk of pneumonia is increased 3- to 10-fold [29,58,60]. The incidence of ventilator-associated pneumonia ranged from 8% to 28% [58,61]. Ventilator-associated pneumonia is defined as pneumonia occurring >48 h after endotracheal intubation [62]. Some use the term hospital-acquired pneumonia to denote any pneumonia developing in the hospital (including ventilator-associated pneumonia) and others exclude ventilator-associated pneumonia from the hospital-acquired pneumonia designation [62]. Therefore, the comparability of the literature is complicated by inconsistent usage of the terms. Four of the studies in this review used the term "ventilator-associated pneumonia" [37,42,43,55] and one study used the term "hospital-acquired infection" [63]. The difference between successful or unsuccessful weaning from mechanical ventilation showed differences in the incidences of pneumonia, but this relies on only one study and hence no conclusion can be drawn. From all pneumonia events in hospital, about 60% occur in non-ventilated patients with SCI [64]. The incidence of hospital-acquired pneumonia is low (1.6%) in the non-ventilated general population [65]. These 1.6% correspond to about 22% of all hospital-acquired infections.

4.2.4. Tracheostomy

Tracheostomy seems likely to influence the incidence of pneumonia, but this relies only on one single study [39]. In this study, no statistical significance for the timing of tracheostomy and pneumonia was given. Other studies report that the rates of pneumonia in SCI cannot be reduced by the timing of tracheostomy [66,67]. However, the timing of the tracheostomy within 7 days of entry to ICU is associated with a shorter duration of mechanical ventilation and shorter length of ICU stay [66–68]. A review of patients with trauma in ICU summarized the impact of timing of tracheostomy on pneumonia, and it reported that some studies found a reduction in pneumonia but some did not [69].

4.2.5. Dysphagia

Dysphagia seems to be an important variable linked to the incidence of pneumonia, but only a few studies provided data that could be used. The most common cause of death in patients with dysphagia due to neurological disorders is aspiration pneumonia [70,71]. This is defined as an infection caused by the inhalation of oropharyngeal secretions that are colonized by pathogenic bacteria [72]. Generally, 5% to 15% of cases with community-acquired pneumonia are aspiration pneumonia [72,73]. The included studies in this review did not formally consider aspiration pneumonia.

4.2.6. General Aspects

Due to the different compositions of setting, level of injury, mechanical ventilation, tracheostomy, and dysphagia in our sub-analyses, a direct comparison with the general population is difficult.

Generally, to reduce pneumonia incidence, a rapid identification of infected patients and appropriate antimicrobial or other treatment is required [58]. Unfortunately, qualitative influence on incidence such as time since injury, type of bacterial pneumonia or smoking could not be included due to missing details in the studies. In the future, it would be valuable to have more thorough recording of study characteristics with a clear definition of pneumonia type, setting, and description of ventilation or dysphagia to facilitate future meta-analyses.

4.3. Strengths and Limitations

Our search strategy was planned to comprise extensive literature searches of several major electronic databases as well as contact with experts in the field. Despite these searches, we might miss eligible studies, in particular if they are not published in indexed peer-reviewed journals. This might lead to a reporting bias [74]. Our literature search revealed three papers that were unable to be translated, and this constitutes a potential selection bias. Generally, the included studies were conducted in high-income countries, and therefore, the incidence of pneumonia after SCI in low-income countries could not be reflected in this systematic review. Due to the specific patient group and the strictly defined research question, we did not expect a large number of studies for inclusion. The number of included studies in each single sub-analysis was low (Figure 2). We are aware that many of the included studies were interventional studies with multiple inclusion and exclusion criteria and therefore increased potential risk for pneumonia that could bias our outcomes as well, but in this way all types of pneumonia were included to get an overview of the full picture in SCI. For the covariate setting, the acute phase is not a standardized term and therefore the time period was defined differently in the included studies or was not defined at all; this can lead to a mixture of different times post injury. Even if we had already tried to specify potential sources of clinical diversity by defining strict inclusion criteria in the protocol, we still had high heterogeneity according to the statistical I2 test (Figure 2). Most studies reported cumulative incidences, i.e., the number of events divided by the number of participants. Incidence rates (cases with pneumonia divided by the observed person-time) would be a better statistic, but few studies reported the time the persons were at risk. A further important source of clinical heterogeneity can be the insufficient definition of diagnostic criteria for pneumonia in a number of the included studies (Supplementary File S3). Usually, with high diversity in a systematic review, conclusions need to be interpreted with caution or seen as hypotheses. Finally, we relied on the quality and quantity of available published information. Nonetheless, to our knowledge, this is the first attempt at a systematic review of the incidence of pneumonia in SCI.

5. Conclusions

The main finding of this systematic review and meta-regression is that we found large heterogeneity in the reporting of the incidence of pneumonia, and we therefore should be cautious with interpreting the results. Our overall incidence ranged from 0.03 to 7.21 patients with pneumonia per 100 days, with higher incidence in the acute and ICU setting than later after injury. Large longitudinal studies with a standardized reporting of risk factors, pneumonia, and detailed time under observation are needed. Nevertheless, this review showed that pneumonia is still a clinically relevant complication, and special attention to pneumonia prevention should focus on the ICU setting and patients with complete tetraplegia. We need to focus more on regular screening of pulmonary and respiratory muscle function in the ICU and doing what we can to enhance function (e.g., by respiratory muscle training).

Supplementary Materials: The following are available online at https://www.mdpi.com/article/10.3390/jcm11010211/s1, Supplementary File S1: Search Strategy, Supplementary File S2: Risk-of-Bias-tool, Supplementary File S3: Risk-of-Bias assessment summary, Supplementary File S4: List of excluded full texts, Supplementary File S5: Sensitivity analyses with two alternative calculations of the time under risk.

Author Contributions: Conceptualization, A.M.R., G.M. and R.H.; methodology, A.M.R. and R.H.; software, R.H.; validation, A.M.R., R.H. and M.Z.; formal analysis, A.M.R. and S.E.; data curation, R.H., M.Z.; writing—original draft preparation, A.M.R.; writing—review and editing, G.M., S.E., S.C.G., M.Z., M.T.E.H., R.H.; visualization, R.H.; supervision, M.T.E.H.; project administration, A.M.R.; All authors have read and agreed to the published version of the manuscript.

Funding: This research received no external funding.

Institutional Review Board Statement: Not applicable.

Informed Consent Statement: Not applicable.

Data Availability Statement: Detailed information on study data and analysis are available upon request from the corresponding author.

Acknowledgments: We thank the librarian Hildegard Oswald for her very helpful explanations regarding databases and for the literature search.

Conflicts of Interest: The authors declare no conflict of interest.

References

1. Marsolais, E.B.; Boninger, M.L.; McCormick, P.C.; Love, L.; Mackelprang, R.W.; Dalsey, W.C. Respiratory management following spinal cord injury: A clinical practice guideline for health-care professionals. *J. Spinal Cord Med.* **2005**, *28*, 259–293.
2. Wang, A.Y.; Jaeger, R.J.; Yarkony, G.M.; Turba, R.M. Cough in spinal cord injured patients: The relationship between motor level and peak expiratory flow. *Spinal Cord* **1997**, *35*, 299–302. [CrossRef] [PubMed]
3. Lanig, I.S.; Peterson, W.P. The respiratory system in spinal cord injury. *Phys. Med. Rehabil. Clin. N. Am.* **2000**, *11*, 29–43. [CrossRef]
4. Savic, G.; DeVivo, M.J.; Frankel, H.L.; Jamous, M.A.; Soni, B.M.; Charlifue, S. Causes of death after traumatic spinal cord injury-a 70-year British study. *Spinal Cord* **2017**, *55*, 891–897. [CrossRef] [PubMed]
5. Jackson, A.B.; Groomes, T.E. Incidence of respiratory complications following spinal cord injury. *Arch. Phys. Med. Rehabil.* **1994**, *75*, 270–275. [CrossRef]
6. Berlly, M.; Shem, K. Respiratory management during the first five days after spinal cord injury. *J. Spinal Cord Med.* **2007**, *30*, 309–318. [CrossRef] [PubMed]
7. CDC. Causes of Pneumonia. Available online: https://www.cdc.gov/pneumonia/causes.html (accessed on 18 May 2021).

8. Torres, A.; Blasi, F.; Peetermans, W.E.; Viegi, G.; Welte, T. The aetiology and antibiotic management of community-acquired pneumonia in adults in Europe: A literature review. *Eur. J. Clin. Microbiol. Infect. Dis.* **2014**, *33*, 1065–1079. [CrossRef] [PubMed]
9. Welte, T.; Torres, A.; Nathwani, D. Clinical and economic burden of community-acquired pneumonia among adults in Europe. *Thorax* **2012**, *67*, 71–79. [CrossRef] [PubMed]
10. Agostinello, J.; Battistuzzo, C.R.; Batchelor, P.E. Early clinical predictors of pneumonia in critically ill spinal cord injured individuals: A retrospective cohort study. *Spinal Cord* **2019**, *57*, 41–48. [CrossRef] [PubMed]
11. Osterthun, R.; Post, M.W.; van Asbeck, F.W.; van Leeuwen, C.M.; van Koppenhagen, C.F. Causes of death following spinal cord injury during inpatient rehabilitation and the first five years after discharge. A Dutch cohort study. *Spinal Cord* **2014**, *52*, 483–488. [CrossRef]
12. Ahoniemi, E.; Pohjolainen, T.; Kautiainen, H. Survival after spinal cord injury in Finland. *J. Rehabil. Med.* **2011**, *43*, 481–485. [CrossRef] [PubMed]
13. Lidal, I.B.; Snekkevik, H.; Aamodt, G.; Hjeltnes, N.; Biering-Sorensen, F.; Stanghelle, J.K. Mortality after spinal cord injury in Norway. *J. Rehabil. Med.* **2007**, *39*, 145–151. [CrossRef]
14. Weaver, F.M.; Smith, B.; Evans, C.T.; Kurichi, J.E.; Patel, N.; Kapur, V.K.; Burns, S.P. Outcomes of outpatient visits for acute respiratory illness in veterans with spinal cord injuries and disorders. *Am. J. Phys. Med. Rehabil.* **2006**, *85*, 718–726. [CrossRef]
15. Chen, C.F.; Lien, I.N.; Wu, M.C. Respiratory function in patients with spinal cord injuries: Effects of posture. *Paraplegia* **1990**, *28*, 81–86. [CrossRef] [PubMed]
16. Brown, R.; DiMarco, A.F.; Hoit, J.D.; Garshick, E. Respiratory dysfunction and management in spinal cord injury. *Respir. Care* **2006**, *51*, 853–868.
17. Emmi, V. [Guidelines for treatment of pneumonia in intensive care units]. *Infez. Med.* **2005**, 7–17. Available online: https://pubmed.ncbi.nlm.nih.gov/16801748/ (accessed on 18 May 2021).
18. Hayashi, T.; Fujiwara, Y.; Sakai, H.; Kubota, K.; Kawano, O.; Mori, E.; Takao, T.; Masuda, M.; Morishita, Y.; Maeda, T. The time course of dysphagia following traumatic cervical spinal cord injury: A prospective cohort study. *Spinal Cord* **2020**, *58*, 53–57. [CrossRef]
19. Shem, K.; Castillo, K.; Wong, S.; Chang, J. Dysphagia in individuals with tetraplegia: Incidence and risk factors. *J. Spinal Cord Med.* **2011**, *34*, 85–92. [CrossRef]
20. Shem, K.; Castillo, K.; Wong, S.L.; Chang, J.; Kolakowsky-Hayner, S. Dysphagia and respiratory care in individuals with tetraplegia: Incidence, associated factors, and preventable complications. *Top. Spinal Cord Inj. Rehabil.* **2012**, *18*, 15–22. [CrossRef]
21. Martin, N.D.; Marks, J.A.; Donohue, J.; Giordano, C.; Cohen, M.J.; Weinstein, M.S. The mortality inflection point for age and acute cervical spinal cord injury. *J. Trauma* **2011**, *71*, 380–385; discussion 385–386. [CrossRef] [PubMed]
22. Munn, Z.; Moola, S.; Riitano, D.; Lisy, K. The development of a critical appraisal tool for use in systematic reviews addressing questions of prevalence. *Int. J. Health Policy Manag.* **2014**, *3*, 123–128. [CrossRef]
23. Moher, D.; Liberati, A.; Tetzlaff, J.; Altman, D.G. Preferred reporting items for systematic reviews and meta-analyses: The PRISMA statement. *Int. J. Surg.* **2010**, *8*, 336–341. [CrossRef] [PubMed]
24. Stroup, D.F.; Berlin, J.A.; Morton, S.C.; Olkin, I.; Williamson, G.D.; Rennie, D.; Moher, D.; Becker, B.J.; Sipe, T.A.; Thacker, S.B. Meta-analysis of observational studies in epidemiology: A proposal for reporting. Meta-analysis Of Observational Studies in Epidemiology (MOOSE) group. *JAMA* **2000**, *283*, 2008–2012. [CrossRef] [PubMed]
25. Biering-Sørensen, F.; DeVivo, M.; Charlifue, S.; Chen, Y.; New, P.; Noonan, V.; Post, M.; Vogel, L. International spinal cord injury core data set (version 2.0)—including standardization of reporting. *Spinal Cord* **2017**, *55*, 759–764. [CrossRef] [PubMed]
26. CDC. Lesson 3: Measures of Risk; Sectiion 2: Morbidity Frequency Measures. Available online: https://www.cdc.gov/csels/dsepd/ss1978/lesson3/section2.html#:~{}:text=The%20denominator%20of%20an%20incidence,be%20included%20in%20the%20numerator. (accessed on 18 May 2021).
27. Hoy, D.; Brooks, P.; Woolf, A.; Blyth, F.; March, L.; Bain, C.; Baker, P.; Smith, E.; Buchbinder, R. Assessing risk of bias in prevalence studies: Modification of an existing tool and evidence of interrater agreement. *J. Clin. Epidemiol.* **2012**, *65*, 934–939. [CrossRef] [PubMed]
28. Stijnen, T.; Hamza, T.H.; Ozdemir, P. Random effects meta-analysis of event outcome in the framework of the generalized linear mixed model with applications in sparse data. *Stat. Med.* **2010**, *29*, 3046–3067. [CrossRef]
29. Oliveira, J.; Zagalo, C.; Cavaco-Silva, P. Prevention of ventilator-associated pneumonia. *Rev. Port. Pneumol.* **2014**, *20*, 152–161. [CrossRef]
30. Shem, K.; Wong, J.; Dirlikov, B.; Castillo, K. Pharyngeal Dysphagia in Individuals With Cervical Spinal Cord Injury: A Prospective Observational Cohort Study. *Top. Spinal Cord Inj. Rehabil.* **2019**, *25*, 322–330. [CrossRef]
31. Spittal, M.J.; Pirkis, J.; Gurrin, L.C. Meta-analysis of incidence rate data in the presence of zero events. *BMC Med. Res. Methodol.* **2015**, *15*, 42. [CrossRef] [PubMed]
32. Kirkwood, B.R.; Sterne, J.A. *Essential Medical Statistics*; John Wiley & Sons: Hoboken, NJ, USA, 2010.
33. Higgins, J.P.T.; Thompson, S.G.; Deeks, J.J.; Altman, D.G. Measuring inconsistency in meta-analyses. *BMJ* **2003**, *327*, 557–560. [CrossRef] [PubMed]
34. Higgins, J.P.; Thompson, S.G. Quantifying heterogeneity in a meta-analysis. *Stat. Med.* **2002**, *21*, 1539–1558. [CrossRef]
35. Balduzzi, S.; Rücker, G.; Schwarzer, G. How to perform a meta-analysis with R: A practical tutorial. *Evid. Based Ment. Health* **2019**, *22*, 153–160. [CrossRef]

36. Viechtbauer, W. Conducting Meta-Analyses in R with the metafor Package. *J. Stat. Softw.* **2010**, *36*, 1–48. [CrossRef]
37. Garcia-Leoni, M.E.; Moreno, S.; Garcia-Garrote, F.; Cercenado, E. Ventilator-associated pneumonia in long-term ventilator-assisted individuals. *Spinal Cord* **2010**, *48*, 876–880. [CrossRef] [PubMed]
38. Medee, B.; Girard, R.; Loukili, A.; Loiseau, K.; Tell, L.; Rode, G. Lower respiratory events in seated tracheotomized tetraplegic patients. *Eur. J. Phys. Rehabil. Med.* **2010**, *46*, 37–42. [PubMed]
39. Choi, H.J.; Paeng, S.H.; Kim, S.T.; Lee, K.S.; Kim, M.S.; Jung, Y.T. The Effectiveness of Early Tracheostomy (within at least 10 Days) in Cervical Spinal Cord Injury Patients. *J. Korean Neurosurg. Soc.* **2013**, *54*, 220–224. [CrossRef] [PubMed]
40. Citak, M.; Suero, E.M.; Backhaus, M.; Aach, M.; Godry, H.; Meindl, R.; Schildhauer, T.A. Risk factors for heterotopic ossification in patients with spinal cord injury: A case-control study of 264 patients. *Spine* **2012**, *37*, 1953–1957. [CrossRef] [PubMed]
41. Fenton, J.J.; Warner, M.L.; Lammertse, D.; Charlifue, S.; Martinez, L.; Dannels-McClure, A.; Kreider, S.; Pretz, C. A comparison of high vs. standard tidal volumes in ventilator weaning for individuals with sub-acute spinal cord injuries: A site-specific randomized clinical trial. *Spinal Cord* **2016**, *54*, 234–238. [CrossRef]
42. Fussenich, W.; Hirschfeld Araujo, S.; Kowald, B.; Hosman, A.; Auerswald, M.; Thietje, R. Discontinuous ventilator weaning of patients with acute SCI. *Spinal Cord* **2018**, *56*, 461–468. [CrossRef]
43. Hatton, G.E.; Mollett, P.J.; Du, R.E.; Wei, S.; Korupolu, R.; Wade, C.E.; Adams, S.D.; Kao, L.S. High tidal volume ventilation is associated with ventilator-associated pneumonia in acute cervical spinal cord injury. *J. Spinal Cord Med.* **2020**, *44*, 775–781. [CrossRef] [PubMed]
44. Ito, Y.; Sugimoto, Y.; Tomioka, M.; Kai, N.; Tanaka, M. Does high dose methylprednisolone sodium succinate really improve neurological status in patient with acute cervical cord injury?: A prospective study about neurological recovery and early complications. *Spine* **2009**, *34*, 2121–2124. [CrossRef]
45. Kamiya, K.; Koda, M.; Furuya, T.; Kato, K.; Takahashi, H.; Sakuma, T.; Inada, T.; Ota, M.; Maki, S.; Okawa, A.; et al. Neuroprotective therapy with granulocyte colony-stimulating factor in acute spinal cord injury: A comparison with high-dose methylprednisolone as a historical control. *Eur. Spine J.* **2015**, *24*, 963–967. [CrossRef]
46. McKinley, W.; Meade, M.A.; Kirshblum, S.; Barnard, B. Outcomes of early surgical management versus late or no surgical intervention after acute spinal cord injury. *Arch. Phys. Med. Rehabil.* **2004**, *85*, 1818–1825. [CrossRef] [PubMed]
47. McKinley, W.O.; Tewksbury, M.A.; Godbout, C.J. Comparison of medical complications following nontraumatic and traumatic spinal cord injury. *J. Spinal Cord Med.* **2002**, *25*, 88–93. [CrossRef]
48. Patel, A.; Smith, H.E.; Radcliff, K.; Yadlapalli, N.; Vaccaro, A.R. Odontoid fractures with neurologic deficit have higher mortality and morbidity. *Clin. Orthop. Relat. Res.* **2012**, *470*, 1614–1620. [CrossRef]
49. Raab, A.M.; Krebs, J.; Perret, C.; Michel, F.; Hopman, M.T.; Mueller, G. Maximum Inspiratory Pressure is a Discriminator of Pneumonia in Individuals With Spinal-Cord Injury. *Respir. Care* **2016**, *61*, 1636–1643. [CrossRef]
50. Smith, B.M.; Evans, C.T.; Kurichi, J.E.; Weaver, F.M.; Patel, N.; Burns, S.P. Acute respiratory tract infection visits of veterans with spinal cord injuries and disorders: Rates, trends, and risk factors. *J. Spinal Cord Med.* **2007**, *30*, 355–361. [CrossRef]
51. Stillman, M.D.; Barber, J.; Burns, S.; Williams, S.; Hoffman, J.M. Complications of Spinal Cord Injury Over the First Year after Discharge from Inpatient Rehabilitation. *Arch. Phys. Med. Rehabil.* **2017**, *98*, 1800–1805. [CrossRef] [PubMed]
52. Street, J.T.; Noonan, V.K.; Cheung, A.; Fisher, C.G.; Dvorak, M.F. Incidence of acute care adverse events and long-term health-related quality of life in patients with TSCI. *Spine J.* **2015**, *15*, 923–932. [CrossRef]
53. Unsal-Delialioglu, S.; Kaya, K.; Sahin-Onat, S.; Kulakli, F.; Culha, C.; Ozel, S. Fever during rehabilitation in patients with traumatic spinal cord injury: Analysis of 392 cases from a national rehabilitation hospital in Turkey. *J. Spinal Cord Med.* **2010**, *33*, 243–248. [CrossRef]
54. Wahman, K.; Nilsson Wikmar, L.; Chlaidze, G.; Joseph, C. Secondary medical complications after traumatic spinal cord injury in Stockholm, Sweden: Towards developing prevention strategies. *J. Rehabil. Med.* **2019**, *51*, 513–517. [CrossRef]
55. Younan, D.; Lin, E.; Griffin, R.; Vanlandingham, S.; Waters, A.; Harrigan, M.; Pittet, J.F.; Kerby, J.D. Early Trauma-Induced Coagulopathy is Associated with Increased Ventilator-Associated Pneumonia in Spinal Cord Injury Patients. *Shock* **2016**, *45*, 502–505. [CrossRef]
56. Yu, W.K.; Ko, H.K.; Ho, L.I.; Wang, J.H.; Kou, Y.R. Synergistic impact of acute kidney injury and high level of cervical spinal cord injury on the weaning outcome of patients with acute traumatic cervical spinal cord injury. *Injury* **2015**, *46*, 1317–1323. [CrossRef]
57. Vitaz, T.W.; McIlvoy, L.; Raque, G.H.; Spain, D.A.; Shields, C.B. Development and implementation of a clinical pathway for spinal cord injuries. *J. Spinal Disord.* **2001**, *14*, 271–276. [CrossRef]
58. Chastre, J.; Fagon, J.Y. Ventilator-associated pneumonia. *Am. J. Respir. Crit. Care Med.* **2002**, *165*, 867–903. [CrossRef] [PubMed]
59. Berlowitz, D.J.; Tamplin, J. Respiratory muscle training for cervical spinal cord injury. *Cochrane Database Syst. Rev.* **2013**, *7*, CD008507. [CrossRef]
60. NNIS System. National Nosocomial Infections Surveillance (NNIS) System Report, Data Summary from January 1990–May 1999, issued June 1999. A report from the NNIS System. *Am. J. Infect. Control* **1999**, *27*, 520–532.
61. Bassetti, M.; Taramasso, L.; Giacobbe, D.R.; Pelosi, P. Management of ventilator-associated pneumonia: Epidemiology, diagnosis and antimicrobial therapy. *Expert Rev. Anti-Infect. Ther.* **2012**, *10*, 585–596. [CrossRef] [PubMed]

62. Kalil, A.C.; Metersky, M.L.; Klompas, M.; Muscedere, J.; Sweeney, D.A.; Palmer, L.B.; Napolitano, L.M.; O'Grady, N.P.; Bartlett, J.G.; Carratalà, J.; et al. Management of Adults with Hospital-acquired and Ventilator-associated Pneumonia: 2016 Clinical Practice Guidelines by the Infectious Diseases Society of America and the American Thoracic Society. *Clin. Infect. Dis.* **2016**, *63*, e61–e111. [CrossRef] [PubMed]
63. Evans, C.T.; Lavela, S.L.; Weaver, F.M.; Priebe, M.; Sandford, P.; Niemiec, P.; Miskevics, S.; Parada, J.P. Epidemiology of hospital-acquired infections in veterans with spinal cord injury and disorder. *Infect. Control Hosp. Epidemiol.* **2008**, *29*, 234–242. [CrossRef] [PubMed]
64. Magill, S.S.; Edwards, J.R.; Bamberg, W.; Beldavs, Z.G.; Dumyati, G.; Kainer, M.A.; Lynfield, R.; Maloney, M.; McAllister-Hollod, L.; Nadle, J.; et al. Multistate point-prevalence survey of health care-associated infections. *N. Engl. J. Med.* **2014**, *370*, 1198–1208. [CrossRef]
65. Giuliano, K.K.; Baker, D.; Quinn, B. The epidemiology of nonventilator hospital-acquired pneumonia in the United States. *Am. J. Infect. Control* **2018**, *46*, 322–327. [CrossRef] [PubMed]
66. Galeiras Vazquez, R.; Rascado Sedes, P.; Mourelo Farina, M.; Montoto Marques, A.; Ferreiro Velasco, M.E. Respiratory management in the patient with spinal cord injury. *BioMed Res. Int.* **2013**, *2013*, 168757. [CrossRef] [PubMed]
67. Flanagan, C.D.; Childs, B.R.; Moore, T.A.; Vallier, H.A. Early Tracheostomy in Patients with Traumatic Cervical Spinal Cord Injury Appears Safe and May Improve Outcomes. *Spine* **2018**, *43*, 1110–1116. [CrossRef]
68. Ganuza, J.R.; Forcada, A.G.; Gambarrutta, C.; Buigues, E.D.D.L.L.; Gonzalez, V.E.M.; Fuentes, F.P.; Luciani, A.A. Effect of technique and timing of tracheostomy in patients with acute traumatic spinal cord injury undergoing mechanical ventilation. *J. Spinal Cord Med.* **2011**, *34*, 76–84. [CrossRef]
69. Arabi, Y.; Haddad, S.; Shirawi, N.; Al Shimemeri, A. Early tracheostomy in intensive care trauma patients improves resource utilization: A cohort study and literature review. *Crit. Care* **2004**, *8*, R347–R352. [CrossRef] [PubMed]
70. Ding, C.; Yang, Z.; Wang, J.; Liu, X.; Cao, Y.; Pan, Y.; Han, L.; Zhan, S. Prevalence of Pseudomonas aeruginosa and antimicrobial-resistant Pseudomonas aeruginosa in patients with pneumonia in mainland China: A systematic review and meta-analysis. *Int. J. Infect. Dis.* **2016**, *49*, 119–128. [CrossRef]
71. Bath, P.M.; Lee, H.S.; Everton, L.F. Swallowing therapy for dysphagia in acute and subacute stroke. *Cochrane Database Syst. Rev.* **2018**, *10*, Cd000323. [CrossRef] [PubMed]
72. Marik, P.E. Aspiration pneumonitis and aspiration pneumonia. *N. Engl. J. Med.* **2001**, *344*, 665–671. [CrossRef] [PubMed]
73. Rodriguez, A.E.; Restrepo, M.I. New perspectives in aspiration community acquired Pneumonia. *Expert Rev. Clin. Pharmacol.* **2019**, *12*, 991–1002. [CrossRef] [PubMed]
74. The Cochrane Collaboration. *Cochrane Handbook for Systematic Reviews of Interventions, Updated October 2019*, 2nd ed.; Wiley-Blackwell: Hoboken, NJ, USA, 2019.

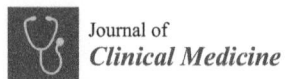

Article

Epidemiological Characterization and the Impact of Healthcare-Associated Pneumonia in Patients Admitted in a Northern Portuguese Hospital

Lucía Méndez [1,2,*], Pedro Castro [3], Jorge Ferreira [1] and Cátia Caneiras [2,4,5]

1. Pneumology Department, Centro Hospitalar de Entre Douro e Vouga, 4520-221 Santa Maria da Feira, Portugal; jorge.ferreira@chedv.min-saude.pt
2. EnviHealthMicro Lab, Microbiology Research Laboratory on Environmental Health, Institute of Environmental Health (ISAMB), Faculty of Medicine, Universidade de Lisboa, 1649-028 Lisboa, Portugal; ccaneiras@medicina.ulisboa.pt
3. Intensive Care Unit, Centro Hospitalar de Entre Douro e Vouga, 4520-221 Santa Maria da Feira, Portugal; pedro.castro@chedv.min-saude.pt
4. Institute of Preventive Medicine and Public Health, Faculty of Medicine, Universidade de Lisboa, 1649-028 Lisboa, Portugal
5. Microbiology and Immunology Department, Faculty of Pharmacy, Universidade de Lisboa, 1649-003 Lisboa, Portugal
* Correspondence: lucia.gonzalez@chedv.min-saude.pt

Abstract: Pneumonia is one of the main causes of hospitalization and mortality. It's the fourth leading cause of death worldwide. Healthcare-associated infections are the most frequent complication of healthcare and affect hundreds of millions of patients around the world, although the actual number of patients affected is unknown due to the difficulty of reliable data. The main goal of this manuscript is to describe the epidemiological characteristics of patients admitted with pneumonia and the impact of healthcare-associated pneumonia (HCAP) in those patients. It is a quantitative descriptive study with retrospective analysis of the clinical processes of 2436 individuals for 1 year (2018) with the diagnosis of pneumonia. The individuals with ≤5 years old represented 10.4% ($n = 253$) and ≥65 were 72.6% ($n = 1769$). 369 cases resulted in death, which gives a sample lethality rate of 15.2%. The severity and mortality index were not sensitive to the death event. We found 30.2% ($n = 735$) individuals with HCAP and 0.41% ($n = 59$) with ventilator-associated pneumonia (VAP). In only 59 individuals (2.4%) the agent causing pneumonia was isolated. The high fatality rate obtained shows that pneumonia is a major cause of death in vulnerable populations. Moreover, HCAP is one of the main causes of hospital admissions from pneumonia and death and the most pneumonias are treated empirically. Knowledge of the epidemiology characterization of pneumonia, especially associated with healthcare, is essential to increase the skills of health professionals for the prevention and efficient treatment of pneumonia.

Keywords: pneumonia; healthcare-associated pneumonia; epidemiology; hospitalization; *Klebsiella pneumoniae*; gram-negative; Portugal

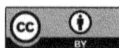

1. Introduction

Pneumonia, along with other lower respiratory tract infections, is the fourth leading cause of death worldwide, accounting for over 4 million deaths per year [1,2]. At the European Union, pneumonia remains the most frequent cause of death from infection, especially in the elderly [3]. In Portugal, pneumonia is one of the main causes of hospitalization and mortality. In 2018, about 40,345 patients were hospitalized with the diagnosis of pneumonia and the associated mortality rate was 20.3% [4].

Nosocomial infections are infections acquired by a patient during healthcare that did not have it or was not incubating it at the time of admission [5]. They constitute the most frequent complication of health care, but the actual number of patients affected is unknown due to the difficulty of reliable data [6]. These infections increase hospital stay, dysfunctions and promote greater resistance of microorganisms to antimicrobials. Healthcare-associated pneumonia (HCAP) includes any patient who was hospitalized in an acute care hospital for two or more days within 90 days of infection; resided in a nursing home or long-term care facility; received recent intravenous antibiotic therapy, chemotherapy, or wound care within the past 30 days of the current infection; attended a hospital or hemodialysis clinic; or lives with a family member infected with a multidrug resistant organism [7,8]. Within HCAP we find the pneumonia acquired by the Hospital (HAP) and the pneumonia associated with the respirator (VAP). HAP is a pneumonia that occurs 48 h or more after admission which was not incubating at the time of admission [7–9]. The definition of VAP is a type of pneumonia acquired in hospitals that occurs more than 48 h after endotracheal intubation. It can be more precisely classified as early onset (until the first 96 h of mechanical ventilation and late onset (more than 96 h after initiation of mechanical ventilation [8,9].

In Portugal, the epidemiological and clinical evidence available is focused on community-acquired pneumonia (CAP) [10–17] at global and regional level in mainland Portugal [18], on CAP and influenza hospitalizations [11,19] and, recently on organizing pneumonia due to COVID-19 [20–22]. No studies have focused specifically on HCAP. In fact, epidemiological data to characterize HCAP are scarce and difficult to obtain, despite the relevance for the scientific knowledge and for prevention and therapeutic optimizing of HCAP. The purpose of this manuscript is to describe the epidemiological characteristics of patients admitted with pneumonia and to evaluate the impact of HCAP within the universe of patients admitted with pneumonia.

2. Materials and Methods

This manuscript describes a descriptive and quantitative study of all individuals hospitalised for pneumonia in a secondary care hospital in northern Portugal during 2018. All individuals admitted to the hospital from 1 January 2018 to 31 December 2018, with the diagnosis of pneumonia, were included. All hospital admission wards were considered. Epidemiological and clinical variables were analysed, namely: age, gender, pathogenic agent isolated, nosocomial pneumonia, severity index and mortality.

The individuals included in the sample were classified as pneumonia, according to the Homogeneous Diagnostic Groups (HDG), according to the All Patient Refined DRGs (APR-DRG) which is a classification system for patients admitted to acute hospitals that incorporate severity of illness. In order to make this grouping, the International Classification of Diseases 9th Clinical Modification of Review (CIE-9-CM) is used in Portugal [23]. Considering the differences in patients with respect to the severity of the disease and the risk of mortality, this diagnostic grouping allows subdivision into subclasses according to these factors. The severity of the disease is understood as an extension of physiological decompensation or loss of organic function and is subclassified as 4 (1: Minor, 2: Moderate, 3: Major and 4: Extreme). The risk of mortality is understood as the patient's probability of death and is subdivided into 4 subclasses (1: Minor, 2: Moderate, 3: Major and 4: Extreme) [24,25].

The classification of the HCAP used was based on the Consensus Document on Nosocomial Pneumonia [5]. The guarantee of confidentiality of the information and the anonymity of the participants was a concern in this study, so that in the data collection and analysis process, there was no element that could identify the individuals in the sample. The study was conducted according to the guidelines of the Declaration of Helsinki, and approved by the Ethics Committee of Centro Hospitalar de Entre Douro e Vouga (protocol code CA-102/2020-0t_MP/AC, 24 April 2020).

3. Results

Between 1 January 2018 and 31 December 2018 were hospitalized 17,176 individuals. Of these, were admitted with the diagnosis of pneumonia 2436 individuals, representing 14.18% of the total number of individuals admitted in that year.

3.1. Epidemiological Characterization

The occurrence of the episodes were more frequent during the coldest months with a total of 61.78% (Autumn: 19.58%, $n = 477$) and Winter: 42.20%, $n = 1028$) than during the more temperate months 38.21% (Spring: 21.84%, $n = 532$) and Summer: 16.38%, $n = 399$). In the sample we found 51.8% ($n = 1262$) men and the mean age was 68.8 ± 27.6 years and median 79 years. Of these 11.9% ($n = 292$) were children of whom 10.38% ($n = 253$) were 5 years old or younger. For individuals over 65 years of age, this corresponds to 72.62% ($n = 1769$) of the sample.

The average length of stay was 10.1 ± 7.2 days, the minimum length of stay was 1 day and the maximum length was 81 days. Of the individuals studied 369 resulted in death, which gives a lethality rate of 15.15% (CI 95%; 13.59–16.67). Among the dead individuals we found 0.04% (CI 95%; 195.72–195.80) ($n = 1$) <5 years and 11.08% (CI 95%; 87.99–111.81) ($n = 270$) >65 years which detailed frequency is presented at Figure 1. The individuals were classified acco-rding to the severity and mortality risk index, following the criteria of the Diagnosis Related Groups (DRG) [25] as it is shown in Table 1.

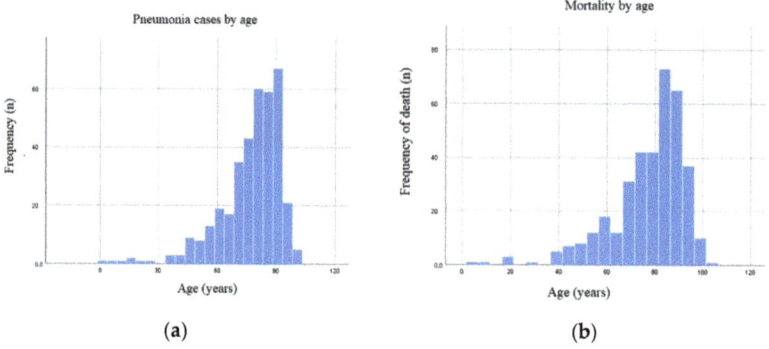

Figure 1. Number of cases of pneumonia (**a**) and mortality (**b**) frequency distributed by age.

Table 1. Classification according to the severity and mortality rates that follows the DRG criteria [25].

Index	Severity (*n*)	%	Mortality Risk (*n*)	%
1	286	11,74	445	18.27
2	530	21.76	386	15.85
3	1363	55.92	1092	44.83
4	252	10.34	508	20.85
Unclassified	5	0.21	5	0.21

To determine the degree of specificity and sensitivity of the severity and mortality rates in relation to death prediction, the Receiver Operating Characteristic curves (ROC curves) were performed and analyzed, as can be seen in Figure 2.

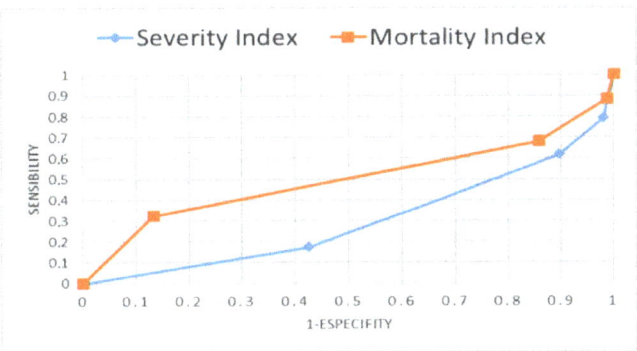

Figure 2. ROC curves of the severity and mortality index as a predictive factor for the occurrence of death.

3.2. Microbiological and HCAP Characterization

At only 59 of the individuals the agents causing pneumonia were isolated, which constitutes 2.42% of the total sample. At 39.28% ($n = 22$) of these isolations the Gram-negative pathogen *Klebsiella pneumoniae* was identified (Figure 3). *Pseudomonas aeruginosa* ($n = 8$) was the second most frequently isolated microorganism.

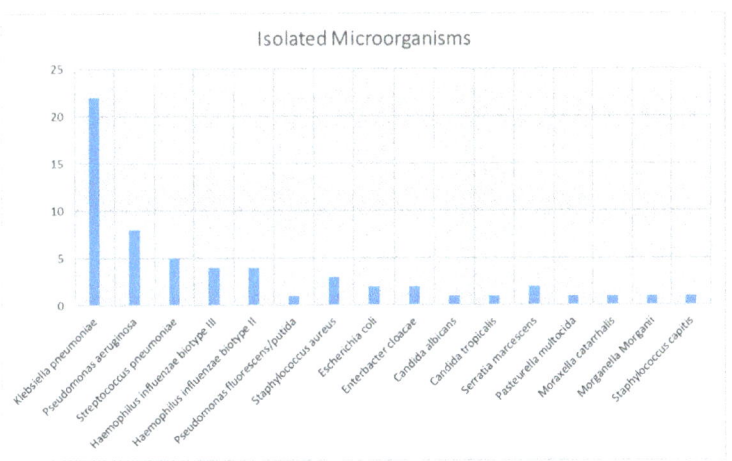

Figure 3. Identification of the microorganisms isolated in respiratory samples.

Considering the 2436 individuals studied with pneumonia, 30.17% ($n = 735$) of their pneumonia were associated with health care. Within these individuals, it was found that in 0.41% ($n = 10$) the pneumonia was associated with mechanical ventilation (VAP) and in 7.92% ($n = 193$) of the cases the pneumonic episode started during the current hospitalization (HAP). Data is shown in Figure 4. Of the 735 individuals with HCAP, 153 died, which is 6.28% of mortality considering all patients with pneumonia, 20.82% of mortality considering the HCAP classification and 41.46% of the total of deaths at hospital at the same period.

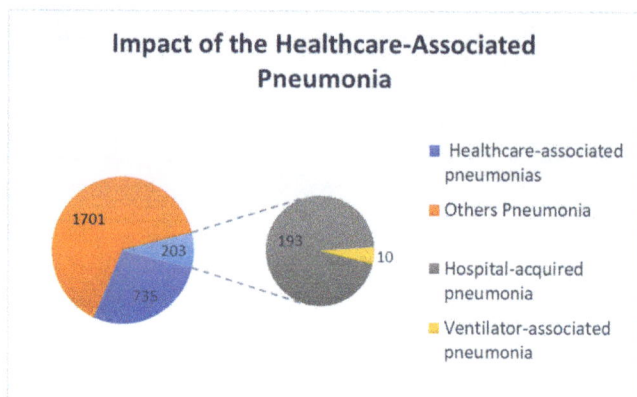

Figure 4. Impact of Healthcare-Associated Pneumonia. This figure represents the number of individuals with HCAP, HAP and VAP, in relation to the total number of individuals admitted for pneumonia.

Mortality was also analysed for each of the different types of nosocomial pneumonia and related to gender. Of the total number of individuals affected by VAP 0.69% ($n = 7$) in relation to the total sample died, being 0.16% ($n = 4$) males and 0.12% ($n = 3$) females. In relation to individuals with HAP, there were 1.72% ($n = 42$), being 0.78% ($n = 19$) males and 0.94% ($n = 23$) females. The rest of the nosocomial pneumonias fell under HCAP and we found that 6.28% ($n = 153$) died during hospitalisation, with 2.91% ($n = 71$) being male and 3.37% ($n = 82$) being female. These data are shown in Table 2.

Table 2. Classification of the types of nosocomial pneumonia and mortality rate, in total number and discriminated by gender and type of pneumonia considering the total of individuals with pneumonia ($n = 2436$).

Pneumonia	Individuals n (%)	Mortality n (%)		
		Total	Male	Female
VAP	10 (0.41)	7 (0.29)	4 (0.16)	3 (0.12)
HAP	193 (7.92)	42 (1.72)	19 (0.78)	23 (0.94)
HCAP	532 (21.84)	104 (4.27)	48 (1.98)	56 (2.30)
Total	735 (30.17)	153 (6.28)	71 (2.91)	82 (3.37)

4. Discussion

The main goal of this study was to characterize the epidemiological and clinical characteristics of the patients admitted with pneumonia at a secondary care hospital in Portugal and to evaluate the impact of HCAP. To the best of authors knowledge, it is the first study focused on HCAP in Portugal.

Pneumonic episodes can occur at any time of the year, they have a greater incidence in the coldest months, especially in winter. The colder air acts as an irritant to the airways, which facilitates the installation and multiplication of infectious agents, and during the colder seasons, people tend to stay longer in closed environments, which favors the propagation of infectious agents among people [26,27]. The gender of individuals is not a predisposing factor for pneumonia, affecting both genders equally. The days of hospital admission obtained in our study corresponds to the average number of days of admission by pneumonia in Portugal [28–30]. Of relevance, the most vulnerable population with the highest associated risk of pneumonia is almost the entire sample (over 65 and 5 years old or younger), so being very young or elderly can be a risk factor for pneumonia. Moreover, we demonstrated an age-dependency on the pneumoniae frequency and mortality.

The health system is fundamental for the success of the treatment and prevention of pneumonia. Moreover, it is essential to ensure access to vaccination for vulnerable populations, as well as to encourage healthy lifestyles, with adequate nutrition and, above all, to encourage breastfeeding in children. The characteristics of our current societies, such as increased environmental pollution and overcrowding, may be aggravating factors for the increase of pneumonic episodes in vulnerable individuals, as well as the increased life expectancy in developed countries [2]. Healthcare-associated pneumonia (HCAP) has been introduced as an entity in the ATS/IDSA guidelines update from 2005 [31] and still is a controversy concept, especially in Europe [32–34] considering the difficulty to identify predictors for such risk [35].

Mortality from pneumonia is improving in most EU countries, however substantial variation in trends remains between countries and Portugal was excluded due to missing data. [36]. The mortality rate obtained in our study (20.82% of mortality considering the HCAP classification) is similar to previous studies on CAP mortality (20.4%, 2000–2009) [17] and total pneumonia (20.3%, 2018) in Portugal [4] but significantly lower when compared to the data reported in 2015 (57.7%) [3]. Some factors that occurred in the last years in Portugal may have helped reduce this rate. In July 2015, the 23-valent pneumococcal polysaccharide (BPPV23) vaccine was included in the National Vaccination Plan [37,38]. Coincidentally, in 2013 the priority health program was created: Program for the Prevention and Control of Infections and Antimicrobial Resistance (PPCIRA), which aims to reduce the rate of infection associated with health care and promote the correct use of antimicrobials [39]. This mortality rate was particularly worrying in the elderly population, in line with a national study that have concluded that patients older than 75 years and comorbidities contribute decisively to the risk of dying from pneumonia in the hospital [40].

Nosocomial pneumonias have a major impact on hospital admissions, constituting a significant number in relation to the total number of complicated pneumonias requiring hospital admission, with a high risk of death from pneumonia [6]. This implies high health and human costs for hospitals. The quality and safety of care provided in hospitals must be a priority for national healthcare systems. Worryingly, most pneumonia (>95%) are treated empirically considering that only in few situations the infectious agent is isolated. At the top of the list of isolations we find *Klebsiella pneumoniae*, which can indicate that the trend of respiratory isolations has changed in the last years and we can highlight the increase of relevance of Gram-negative microorganisms [41]. However, this results should be interpreted with caution regarding that only 2% of the clinical situations have a microorganism identified.

Of relevance, pneumonia has represented >40% of the total of deaths at the hospital at the same period, highlighting the need to implement more studies on HCAP epidemiology and clinical burden. Previous studies highlighted that room for improvement in antibiotic prescription in Healthcare-Associated Pneumonia currently remains and that new strategies for a better use of the adopted tools and definition of new antimicrobial stewardship initiatives are needed to improve compliance to recommendations [42]. In fact, local guidelines and recommendations to treat common infectious diseases are a cornerstone of most Antimicrobial Stewardship programs [43]. More precise instruments are needed to heighten clinicians' index of suspicion for treating probable resistant pathogens with appropriate empirical antibiotic choices [42]. Furthermore, an effective surveillance system to provide quality data and improve the monitoring and epidemiologic characterization of Healthcare Associated infections should be evaluated and implemented [44–48].

The Portuguese health institutions code patients with the severity and risk of mortality rates. However, at the clinical level they are not good predictive indicators for the event of death. Their use is more relevant for the management teams of healthcare institutions and standard indices such as Pneumonia severity index or CURB 65, which are suggested by guidelines for pneumonia from American Thoracic Society and Infectious Diseases Society of America [49] are not currently used.

One limitation that this study is the absence of classification of all types of pneumonia that could give us more detailed information about the causes that determine complicated pneumonia that needs hospital admission. Another limitation found is the absence of the antibiotherapy used, which would give us the therapeutic tendency used in the empirical treatment of pneumonia. Overall mortality should be higher in patients who attended a hospital or hemodialysis clinic or received intravenous chemotherapy in the 30 days before pneumonia, and among patients who resided in a nursing home or long-term-care facility [34]. Given the focus on HCAP, information on the Healthcare setting frequented by these patients would be useful, as well as the delay of onset of the HCAP and unfortunately was not available. However, this study provides a robust epidemiological characterization of pneumonia, especially HCAP. To the best authors knowledge this is the first study in Portugal that addressed HCAP epidemiology and clinical burden. Future research is needed to increase knowledge about other types of pneumonia and the relation with causative agents and the treatment used, to better understand the impact that pneumonia on the hospital population.

5. Conclusions

This manuscript highlight that pneumonia constitute a high risk of mortality for vulnerable populations and is one of the leading causes of hospital admission. The impact of HCAP alerts us to the critical action of infection prevention and control measures in hospitals and should incentive the increase of scientific studies in this crucial area. Reducing the incidence of pneumonia in general and HCAP in particular, will allow an significative improvement in the quality and safety of patient healthcare.

Author Contributions: Conceptualization, L.M. and C.C.; Formal analysis, L.M. and P.C.; Investigation, L.M. and J.F.; Methodology, L.M.; Supervision, C.C.; Writing—original draft, L.M.; Writing—review & editing, L.M., P.C., J.F. and C.C. All authors have read and agreed to the published version of the manuscript.

Funding: This research received no external funding.

Institutional Review Board Statement: The study was conducted according to the guidelines of the Declaration of Helsinki, and approved by the Ethics Committee of Centro Hospitalar de Entre Douro e Vouga (protocol code CA-102/2020-0t_MP/AC, 24 April 2020).

Informed Consent Statement: The research has been based on the retrospective analysis of clinical data so the informed consent statement is not required.

Conflicts of Interest: The authors declare no conflict of interest.

References

1. Nacional Institute of Health and Care Excellence. Pneumonia in adults: Diagnosis and Pneumonia in adults: Diagnosis and management. Published: 3 December 2014. Available online: www.nice.org.uk/guidance/cg191 (accessed on 2 February 2019).
2. Fórum Internacional de Sociedades Respiratórias. O Impacto Global da Doença Respiratória—Segunda Edição—2017. Available online: https://www.who.int/gard/publications/The_Global_Impact_of_Respiratory_Disease_POR.pdf (accessed on 10 March 2019).
3. OECD/European Union. Health at a Glance: Europe 2018: State of Health in the EU Cycle, OECD Publishing, Paris/European Union, Brussels 2018. Available online: https://doi.org/10.1787/health_glance_eur-2018-en (accessed on 12 April 2019).
4. Carvalheira Santos, A. 13º Relatorio do Observatorio Nacional de Doenas Respiratorias 2016/2017. Available online: https://www.ondr.pt/files/Relatorio_ONDR_2018.pdf (accessed on 20 April 2019).
5. Froes, F.; Paiva, J.A.; Amaro, P.; Baptista, J.P.; Brum, G.; Bento, H.; Duarte, P.; Dias, C.S.; Gloria, C.; Estrada, H.; et al. Consensus document on nosocomial pneumonia. *Rev. Port. Pneumol.* **2007**, *13*, 419–486. [CrossRef]
6. Kyu, H.H.; Abate, D.; Abate, K.H.; Abay, S.M.; Abbafati, C.; Abbasi, N.; Abbastabar, H.; Abd-Allah, F.; Abdela, J.; Abdelalim, A.; et al. Global, regional, and national disability-adjusted life-years (DALYs) for 359 diseases and injuries and healthy life expectancy (HALE) for 195 countries and territories, 1990–2017: A systematic analysis for the Global Burden of Disease Study 2017. *Lancet* **2018**, *392*, 1859–1922. [CrossRef]
7. Guimaraes, C.; Lares Santos, C.; Costa, F.; Barata, F. Pneumonia associated with health care versus community acquired pneumonia: Different entities, distinct approaches. *Rev. Port. Pneumol.* **2011**, *17*, 168–171. [CrossRef]

8. Torres, A.; Niederman, M.S.; Chastre, J.; Ewig, S.; Fernandez-Vandellos, P.; Hanberger, H.; Kollef, M.; Li Bassi, G.; Luna, C.M.; Martin-Loeches, I.; et al. International ERS/ESICM/ESCMID/ALAT guidelines for the management of hospital-acquired pneumonia and ventilator-associated pneumonia: Guidelines for the management of hospital-acquired pneumonia (HAP)/ventilator-associated pneumonia (VAP) of the European Respiratory Society (ERS), European Society of Intensive Care Medicine (ESICM), European Society of Clinical Microbiology and Infectious Diseases (ESCMID) and Asociacion Latinoamericana del Torax (ALAT). *Eur. Respir. J.* **2017**, *50*. [CrossRef]
9. Kalil, A.C.; Metersky, M.L.; Klompas, M.; Muscedere, J.; Sweeney, D.A.; Palmer, L.B.; Napolitano, L.M.; O'Grady, N.P.; Bartlett, J.G.; Carratala, J.; et al. Management of Adults with Hospital-acquired and Ventilator-associated Pneumonia: 2016 Clinical Practice Guidelines by the Infectious Diseases Society of America and the American Thoracic Society. *Clin. Infect. Dis.* **2016**, *63*, e61–e111. [CrossRef]
10. Antunes, C.; Pereira, M.; Rodrigues, L.; Organista, D.; Cysneiros, A.; Paula, F.; Nunes, B.; Barbosa, P.; Barbara, C.; Escoval, A.; et al. Hospitalization direct cost of adults with community-acquired pneumonia in Portugal from 2000 to 2009. *Pulmonology* **2020**, *26*, 264–267. [CrossRef]
11. Dias, J.; Correia, A.M.; Queiros, L. Community-acquired pneumonia and influenza hospitalisations in northern Portugal, 2000–2005. *Eurosurveillance* **2007**, *12*, 13–14. [CrossRef] [PubMed]
12. Froes, F. Morbidity and mortality of community-acquired pneumonia in adults in Portugal. *Acta Med. Port.* **2013**, *26*, 644–645. [PubMed]
13. Froes, F.; Diniz, A.; Mesquita, M.; Serrado, M.; Nunes, B. Hospital admissions of adults with community-acquired pneumonia in Portugal between 2000 and 2009. *Eur. Respir. J.* **2013**, *41*, 1141–1146. [CrossRef]
14. Oliveira, A.G. Current management of hospitalized community acquired pneumonia in Portugal. Consensus statements of an expert panel. *Rev. Port. Pneumol.* **2005**, *11*, 243–282.
15. Pessoa, E.; Barbara, C.; Viegas, L.; Costa, A.; Rosa, M.; Nogueira, P. Factors associated with in-hospital mortality from community-acquired pneumonia in Portugal: 2000–2014. *BMC Pulm. Med.* **2020**, *20*, 18. [CrossRef]
16. Oliveira, A.G. Current management of hospitalized community acquired pneumonia in Portugal. Consensus statements of an expert panel. *Rev. Port. Pneumol.* **2006**, *12*, 211–212, author reply 213.
17. Teixeira-Lopes, F.; Cysneiros, A.; Dias, A.; Durao, V.; Costa, C.; Paula, F.; Serrado, M.; Nunes, B.; Diniz, A.; Froes, F. Intra-hospital mortality for community-acquired pneumonia in mainland Portugal between 2000 and 2009. *Pulmonology* **2019**, *25*, 66–70. [CrossRef]
18. Froes, F. Pneumonia in the adult population in continental Portugal—Incidence and mortality in hospitalized patients from 1998 to 2000. *Rev. Port. Pneumol.* **2003**, *9*, 187–194. [CrossRef]
19. Rodrigues, E.; Machado, A.; Silva, S.; Nunes, B. Excess pneumonia and influenza hospitalizations associated with influenza epidemics in Portugal from season 1998/1999 to 2014/2015. *Influenza Other Respir Viruses* **2018**, *12*, 153–160. [CrossRef]
20. Camoes, J.; Lobato, C.T.; Beires, F.; Gomes, E. Legionella and SARS-CoV-2 Coinfection in a Patient With Pneumonia—An Outbreak in Northern Portugal. *Cureus* **2021**, *13*, e12476. [CrossRef] [PubMed]
21. Carvalho, A.; Cunha, R.; Lima, B.A.; Pereira, J.M.; Madureira, A.J. Chest CT imaging features of COVID-19 pneumonia: First radiological insights from Porto, Portugal. *Eur. J. Radiol. Open* **2020**, *7*, 100294. [CrossRef] [PubMed]
22. Méndez, L.; Ferreira, J.; Caneiras, C. *Hafnia alvei* Pneumonia: A Rare Cause of Infection in a Patient with COVID-19. *Microorganisms* **2021**, *9*, 2369. [CrossRef]
23. International Classification of Diseases, Ninth Revision (ICD-9) (2015). Centers for Disease Control and Prevention. Available online: https://www.cdc.gov/nchs/icd/icd9.htm (accessed on 3 April 2019).
24. Agrupador de GDH (Grupos de Diagnósticos Homogéneos) All Patient Refined DRG (Diagnosis Related Groups), Circular Normativa N° 22/2014/DPS/ACSS (2014). Administração Central dos Sistemas de Saúde. Available online: http://www2.acss.min-saude.pt/Default.aspx?TabId=460&language=pt-PT (accessed on 10 April 2019).
25. Fetter, R.B. *Diagnosis Related Groups: A Product Oriented Approach to Hospital Management, Health Systems Management Group*; School of Organization and Management, Yale University: New Haven, CT, USA, 1983.
26. Irizar Aramburu, M.I.; Arrondo Beguiristain, M.A.; Insausti Carretero, M.J.; Mujica Campos, J.; Etxabarri Perez, P.; Ganzarain Gorosabel, R. Epidemiology of community-acquired pneumonia. *Aten Primaria* **2013**, *45*, 503–513. [CrossRef]
27. Saynajakangas, P.; Keistinen, T.; Tuuponen, T. Seasonal fluctuations in hospitalisation for pneumonia in Finland. *Int. J. Circumpolar Health* **2001**, *60*, 34–40. [CrossRef] [PubMed]
28. Direção-Geral da Saúde. Doenças Respiratórias em Números, 2015 Programa Nacional para as Doenças Respiratórias. 2016. Available online: https://www.dgs.pt/estatisticas-de-saude/estatisticas-de-saude/publicacoes/portugal-doencas-respiratorias-em-numeros-2015- (accessed on 2 May 2019).
29. Instituto Nacional de Estatística Portugal. Available online: https://www.ine.pt/xportal/xmain?xpid=INE&xpgid=ine_publicacoes&PUBLICACOESpub_boui=277095050&PUBLICACOESmodo=2&xlang=pt (accessed on 14 May 2019).
30. Menendez, R.; Cremades, M.J.; Martinez-Moragon, E.; Soler, J.J.; Reyes, S.; Perpina, M. Duration of length of stay in pneumonia: Influence of clinical factors and hospital type. *Eur. Respir. J.* **2003**, *22*, 643–648. [CrossRef]
31. American Thoracic Society (ATS); Infectious Diseases Society of America (IDSA). Guidelines for the management of adults with hospital-acquired, ventilator-associated, and healthcareassociated pneumonia. *Am. J. Respir. Crit. Care Med.* **2005**, *171*, 388–416. [CrossRef]

32. Carratala, J.; Mykietiuk, A.; Fernandez-Sabe, N.; Suarez, C.; Dorca, J.; Verdaguer, R.; Manresa, F.; Gudiol, F. Health care-associated pneumonia requiring hospital admission: Epidemiology, antibiotic therapy, and clinical outcomes. *Arch. Intern. Med.* **2007**, *167*, 1393–1399. [CrossRef]
33. Chalmers, J.D.; Taylor, J.K.; Singanayagam, A.; Fleming, G.B.; Akram, A.R.; Mandal, P.; Choudhury, G.; Hill, A.T. Epidemiology, antibiotic therapy, and clinical outcomes in health care-associated pneumonia: A UK cohort study. *Clin. Infect. Dis.* **2011**, *53*, 107–113. [CrossRef]
34. Garcia-Vidal, C.; Viasus, D.; Roset, A.; Adamuz, J.; Verdaguer, R.; Dorca, J.; Gudiol, F.; Carratala, J. Low incidence of multidrug-resistant organisms in patients with healthcare-associated pneumonia requiring hospitalization. *Clin. Microbiol. Infect.* **2011**, *17*, 1659–1665. [CrossRef]
35. Ewig, S.; Welte, T. Adding fuel to the flames? It is time to leave HCAP. *Respir. Med.* **2012**, *106*, 1309–1310. [CrossRef]
36. Marshall, D.C.; Goodson, R.J.; Xu, Y.; Komorowski, M.; Shalhoub, J.; Maruthappu, M.; Salciccioli, J.D. Trends in mortality from pneumonia in the Europe union: A temporal analysis of the European detailed mortality database between 2001 and 2014. *Respir. Res.* **2018**, *19*, 81. [CrossRef] [PubMed]
37. Direção-Geral da Saúde. *Vacinação Contra Infeções por Streptococcus Pneumoniae de Grupos com Risco Acrescido para Doença Invasiva Pneumocócica (DIP)–Adultos (≥18 anos de idade): Norma n° 011/2015, de 23/06/2015, Atualização de 06/11/2015*; DGS: Lisboa, Portugal, 2015.
38. Froes, F.; Diniz, A.; Robalo Cordeiro, C.; Serrado, M.; Ramalho de Almeida, A.; Portuguese Respiratory, S. Consensus document for the prevention of respiratory infections in adults. *Rev. Port. Pneumol.* **2014**, *20*, 111–114. [CrossRef] [PubMed]
39. *Despacho n.° 2902/2013 Programa de Prevenção e Controlo de Infeções e de Resistência aos Antimicrobianos (PPCIRA), pelo Despacho n.° 2902/2013*; Diário da República, 2.ª Série, n.° 38; Imprensa Nacional Casa da Moeda: Lisboa, Portugal, 2013.
40. Hespanhol, V.; Barbara, C. Pneumonia mortality, comorbidities matter? *Pulmonology* **2020**, *26*, 123–129. [CrossRef]
41. Méndez, L.; Pedrosa, A.; Caneiras, C. Growing Growing importance of Gram-negative isolates in respiratory samples. *Eur. Respir. J.* **2020**, *56*, 2027. [CrossRef]
42. Zilberberg, M.D.; Shorr, A.F. Epidemiology of healthcare-associated pneumonia (HCAP). *Semin. Respir. Crit. Care Med.* **2009**, *30*, 10–15. [CrossRef] [PubMed]
43. Cattani, G.; Madia, A.; Arnoldo, L.; Brunelli, L.; Celotto, D.; Grillone, L.; Valent, F.; Castriotta, L.; Pea, F.; Bassetti, M.; et al. Assessment of the impact of clinical recommendations on antibiotic use for CAP and HCAP: Results from an implementation program in an Academic Hospital. *Ann Ig* **2020**, *32*, 344–356. [CrossRef]
44. Behnke, M.; Valik, J.K.; Gubbels, S.; Teixeira, D.; Kristensen, B.; Abbas, M.; van Rooden, S.M.; Gastmeier, P.; van Mourik, M.S.M.; Aspevall, O.; et al. Information technology aspects of large-scale implementation of automated surveillance of healthcare-associated infections. *Clin. Microbiol. Infect.* **2021**, *27* (Suppl. 1), S29–S39. [CrossRef] [PubMed]
45. Duszynska, W.; Rosenthal, V.D.; Szczesny, A.; Zajaczkowska, K.; Fulek, M.; Tomaszewski, J. Device associated -health care associated infections monitoring, prevention and cost assessment at intensive care unit of University Hospital in Poland (2015–2017). *BMC Infect. Dis.* **2020**, *20*, 761. [CrossRef]
46. Hoskins, A.J.; Worth, L.J.; Imam, N.; Johnson, S.A.; Bull, A.L.; Richards, M.J.; Bennett, N.J. Validation of healthcare-associated infection surveillance in smaller Australian hospitals. *J. Hosp. Infect.* **2018**, *99*, 85–88. [CrossRef] [PubMed]
47. Magill, S.S.; Dumyati, G.; Ray, S.M.; Fridkin, S.K. Evaluating Epidemiology and Improving Surveillance of Infections Associated with Health Care, United States. *Emerg. Infect. Dis.* **2015**, *21*, 1537–1542. [CrossRef]
48. Migliara, G.; Di Paolo, C.; Barbato, D.; Baccolini, V.; Salerno, C.; Nardi, A.; Alessandri, F.; Giordano, A.; Tufi, D.; Marinelli, L.; et al. Multimodal surveillance of healthcare associated infections in an intensive care unit of a large teaching hospital. *Ann Ig* **2019**, *31*, 399–413. [CrossRef]
49. Metlay, J.P.; Waterer, G.W.; Long, A.C.; Anzueto, A.; Brozek, J.; Crothers, K.; Cooley, L.A.; Dean, N.C.; Fine, M.J.; Flanders, S.A.; et al. Diagnosis and Treatment of Adults with Community-acquired Pneumonia. An Official Clinical Practice Guideline of the American Thoracic Society and Infectious Diseases Society of America. *Am. J. Respir. Crit. Care Med.* **2019**, *200*, e45–e67. [CrossRef] [PubMed]

MDPI
St. Alban-Anlage 66
4052 Basel
Switzerland
www.mdpi.com

Journal of Clinical Medicine Editorial Office
E-mail: jcm@mdpi.com
www.mdpi.com/journal/jcm

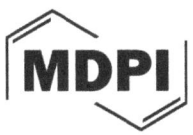

Disclaimer/Publisher's Note: The statements, opinions and data contained in all publications are solely those of the individual author(s) and contributor(s) and not of MDPI and/or the editor(s). MDPI and/or the editor(s) disclaim responsibility for any injury to people or property resulting from any ideas, methods, instructions or products referred to in the content.

www.ingramcontent.com/pod-product-compliance
Lightning Source LLC
LaVergne TN
LVHW070558100526
838202LV00012B/505